What other readers are saying:

"… I have read your book several times and want to keep reading it to get it firmly implanted in my 63 year old head. I can tell you the book is GREAT … I have not taken myself off the 50 mgs of Trazadone yet, but hope to get up the nerve to do so soon. You have a great sense of humor and I can relate to much of what you say."–**Insomniac–Washington**

"… As for your book.....Wonderful! I really enjoyed reading it. You're personal style and insight is very entertaining and informative. You present your ideas in a natural, sincere style that I find refreshing. I can certainly relate to your experiences, and this makes your book especially enjoyable, as opposed to some doctor writing about a topic with no real firsthand knowledge … Overall(,) Great Work! I wish you the best of luck in pursuing this project...and I look forward to buying a first edition!"–**Insominac–Pennsylvania**

"Just finished the book. I really enjoyed it … Most people do not like to read something that sounds too technical or uses too many words that are not understandable … Last night, I slept all night without waking. That was a first time in months."–**Insomniac**

"I have just finished reading your manuscript, and I must say I am impressed, overwhelmed, inspired, envious, and outright awed by your product. As is inescapable for an author, you have bared your heart and soul to your reader, an incredibly unselfish (and frightening) act … What you have done is offered all of us a blueprint for a plan to overcome any behavioral problem we may have … I know the Lord sent me your manuscript for a reason. Isn't it amazing how He uses each one of us?!"–**Anonymous**

"As I read your story I laughed, sympathized, and nodded my head in places (…been there, done that...) … For me the most powerful aspect of your story is the sense of hope it gives to a fellow insomniac."–**Insomniac**

"Just finished the book. It was great … This was well written, funny, compassionate, and uncluttered...Your advice, although I've encountered it before, is certainly based on good research. I've tried much of it at one time or another, with varying results, but I lacked discipline to do it right, as you have done … But you have inspired me to give it another try! And I am very excited. (So excited, I won't fall asleep tonight.)"–**Insomniac-California**

"A heartwarming book that brings hope to chronic insomnia sufferers. John Wiedman shares the pain and triumph of his own personal story. I highly recommend it."–**Mary I. O'Sullivan, President, Quanta Dynamics, Inc.**

"Most insomniacs can list the suspects: stress, anxiety, caffeine, alcohol, etc. Few acknowledge the more common problem: a series of lifestyle choices that frustrate natural biorhythms. *Desperately Seeking Snoozin'* ties it all together, providing the insight and common sense tools to build sleep-promoting behavior and fight the bad habits that keep most people awake."–**Dr. William H. West, Chairman of the Board, Response Oncology. Formerly Senior Researcher at the National Cancer Institute.**

"Overall, I thought it was very good. You mentioned near the end, the importance of having support. Your book (*Desperately Seeking Snoozin'*) provides a pseudo support group to insomnia sufferers ... I would recommend your book to clients/patients etc. for this reason."–**Julia Thomas, Insomnia Clinic of the Methodist Hospital Sleep Disorders Center run by a University of Memphis student with Dr. Kenneth Lichstein as the supervising Clinical Psychologist.**

"John, it's great to speak to someone who can relate to my disorder, I've tried everything in the book that you can think of from medications to locking myself in the bedroom ... your book is great, it's teaching me a lot." **–Insomniac–California**

"I appreciate very much that you have taken so much time to write this book. In particular, you shared your own experience with your readers. I found a lot of similarities between yours and my problems and it really encourage(s) me to believe that there is a cure to my sleeping problems."**– Insomniac–CA**

"Very interesting to read a "firsthand" almost diary account of fellow insomniac's experience. I can identify with a few areas but not the sleeping pills. I've always very much resisted taking drugs and, after your experiences, I'm very glad I did stay away."**–J Ross, Australia**

"I have done extensive work on developing a plan. Out of five nights, I have had two nights where I slept but awoke every hour on the hour, but still felt more rested than I had for a long time. Another night I slept through from 1:30 until 7, which was my wake up time. Last night I abandoned most of my program and as you can imagine, I needed a sleeping pill to get to sleep. So it was a short lesson in discipline, and I am back on track."**–Insomniac–British Columbia**

Desperately Seeking Snoozin'

The Insomnia Cure from Awake to Zzzzz

John Wiedman

Towering Pines Press, Inc.
Memphis Tennessee

DESPERATELY SEEKING SNOOZIN'

THE INSOMNIA CURE

FROM AWAKE TO ZZZZZ

By John Wiedman

Towering Pines Press, Inc.
P. O. Box 17923
Memphis, TN 38187.

First Edition
Publisher: Towering Pines Press, Inc., Memphis, Tennessee
Cover Design and Illustration by Lightbourne Images, copyright © 1998.

Library of Congress Catalog Card Number: 98-090345
ISBN 0-9664189-5-6
Printed in the United States of America

To my wonderful wife, Rhonda, and our three children:
Cary, Brad, and Blake;
and to my mother, Donnie;
and to my lovely granddaughter, Catherine

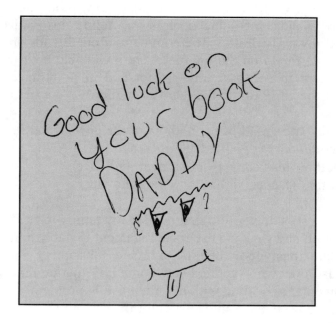

Thanks to Blake for this picture which provided me great encouragement.

Acknowledgments

I would like to thank everyone who gave me the encouragement and feedback necessary to complete this book. Foremost thanks go to my family for their wonderful support, but mainly for letting me monopolize the family computer. Each member of my family lent a hand in contributing to this book. They all had to proofread and/or listen to ideas over and over as to what should and should not be included in the manuscript.

I would like to thank my mother, formerly a registered nurse, for teaching me to always look for an alternative to quick answers from a medicine bottle.

The book would not have been possible without the feedback from my friends, including doctors and fellow insomniacs, who critiqued my early drafts. The comments from friends around the world that I found on the Internet were invaluable both in the encouragement to complete my project and in pointing out those things in the early drafts that somehow didn't quite get the point across.

Thanks, too, to all of the authors of the posts from the Internet whose comments supported the message I was trying to convey. These authors also came from all over the globe.

And finally, special thanks to the following:

- Bill West: who was the first outside my family to read the initial draft and gave me the encouragement to publish my work. Bill graciously took the time to review subsequent changes.
- Linda Pope: who supplied nutritional information that was instrumental in dealing with my night eating problem.
- Cheri Gowen and Paul Delage: for their invaluable contributions.
- Julia Thomas: (a student psychologist at the University of Memphis) for taking the time to give me a professional perspective on my draft.
- Sandman: for allowing me to access information from his Web site.

- John Ross: (a firefighter from South Australia) for suggesting the subtitle.
- Sarah Black: (a good friend) for encouragement as well as her attempts to coach me on the proper use of the English language.

Table of Contents

Author's Note

or

"Is this good enough, Mr. Attorney?"

Although much of this book relates to common sense methods that are meant to help you help yourself, I do not want to be sued. So I am telling you up front...**the purpose of this book is not to take the place of advice from a trained medical professional.** You should always consult with a physician or other competent professional for any of your health problems. I am not a doctor, nor do I have any medical training. Everything in this book is based on my personal experiences. The plan contained in this book worked for me. I cannot assure you that you will have the same results I did.

This book will talk of the ineffectiveness of medications and other aids in treating chronic insomnia. **I am not telling you to stop taking your current medications. Before discontinuing any medication, consult with your doctor for his approval.** If you feel you have developed a dependence on the medication, have your doctor or another qualified medical professional advise you as to the best method to discontinue the use of the medication.

There are several references in the text to taking a hot bath. **If you have problems such as high blood pressure, heart disease, or anything else that exposure to hot water might possibly ex-acerbate, check with your physician first.**

And last, but not least, to the drug manufacturers. The purpose of this book is not to question the effectiveness of your products. Your very own literature will list all of the symptoms and many more that are related in this book. Your disclosures will also state that your medication is recommended for short-term treatment of sleeping problems. As a matter of fact, the last time I talked to one of the pharmacists that worked for a manufacturer of trazodone, he informed me that trazodone was never meant to be used as a sleeping aid. So, think of it this way...this book actually helps your industry inform the public as to the proper use of your sleeping products. And for your support, I thank you.

A Note to Readers

I began writing this book in mid-October, 1997. I had started a program to cure my insomnia the first week in October, and I could already tell that the steps I was taking were working better than I could have ever imagined. I completed my first draft at the end of 1997. I had always felt as though the solution I used to cure my insomnia might be beneficial to others with the same problem. Even with this belief, I had a hard time letting others view my work, as I had never written anything in my life. My family, who had been somewhat skeptical about my writing the book initially, thought I had done a pretty good job. I was still reluctant to let anyone else see the paper. Finally, I broke down and gave a copy to a friend who happens to be both an insomniac and a doctor. I have always had the greatest respect for him and knew that if he liked my manuscript, I might be on to something. I was pleasantly surprised when he gave me some encouragement to have the work published.

I now had the nerve to send the paper to others. I gave three copies to other physician friends and several other copies to people that I knew to have insomnia. I also gave copies to friends and acquaintances who had heard me talking about the book and requested a copy. Additionally, I sent the manuscript to a handful of insomnia sufferers that I found on the Internet who agreed to give me written feedback after reading the paper. One of my concerns when I wrote the book was that others would find the sections dealing with my personal experiences boring. Instead, I discovered that most of the insomniacs found it somewhat fascinating to read about someone who had suffered through some of the same problems they had. Some of the readers had more severe insomnia, some said theirs wasn't as bad, but most saw at least a little of themselves in the book. *I discuss some of their comments in the "Feedback" chapter toward the end of the book.*

On the other hand, I was concerned that the doctors would feel as though I was taking unfair shots at the medical community for the lack of knowledge most primary physicians have had in dealing with insomnia. The feedback from the doctors, or at least the way I interpreted it, was also positive, with some saying they would have no problem recommending the book to their patients.

One of the doctors directed me to an article in the December 24, 1997, edition of The Journal of the American Medical Association pertaining to the use of sleeping pills for chronic insomnia. The following are some highlights from the article:

- Recent estimates are that 10% of the adults in the United States (approximately 25 million people) have chronic insomnia, with the annual cost for its treatment estimated at $10.9 billion. (I have seen estimates as high as $64 billion annually when on-the-job accidents and lost productivity are taken into consideration.)
- Individuals with chronic insomnia report elevated levels of stress, anxiety, depression, and medical illnesses and demonstrate interpersonal and occupational impairments when compared with good sleepers.
- There is a risk factor for the development of major depression when insomnia extends over a one year period.
- Studies indicate that untreated chronic insomnia does not remit with time.
- Medication treatments for insomnia predominate over behavioral ones with the frequency of treatment reflected in the observation that prescription sleeping pills are used by 4% (I have seen other estimates up to 5%) of the population in a given year and 0.4% of the population use sleeping pills for more than a year. (In other articles I have seen estimates that up to 25% of the population in the United States took some sort of chemical to help them sleep in 1996, mainly alcohol and over-the-counter sleep aids.)
- Benzodiazepines are the most common class of medications for treating insomnia with adverse effects including daytime sedation, motor incoordination, and cognitive impairments. Long term use carries the additional risks of physical dependence, withdrawal, and rebound insomnia.

- From 1987-1991, clinicians decreased prescriptions of benzo-diazepines by 30% and increased prescriptions of antidepressants (trazodone hydrochloride, amitriptyline hydrochloride, doxepine hydrochloride) by 100%. There are few studies of antidepressants used as hypnotics, and these medications can have their own adverse effects.
- The National Institutes of Health Consensus Conference on Sleeping Pills and Insomnia in 1984 developed guidelines discouraging the use of sedative hypnotics beyond 4 to 6 weeks because of concerns raised over drug misuse, dependency, withdrawal, and rebound insomnia.

In 1988 Congress created the National Commission on Sleep Disorders Research to conduct a comprehensive study of the status of current knowledge and research on sleep disorders. In January, 1993, the Commission delivered its report, Wake Up America: A National Sleep Alert, to Congress. The report, made available by the National Heart, Lung, and Blood Institute, National Institutes of Health, includes the following findings:

- Frequent or chronic insomnia, estimated to affect more than 60 million Americans, about one in every three adults, is a severe problem for approximately half of those individuals.
- The insomnias cost the United States an estimated $15.4 billion in direct costs alone. Additional costs to society for such consequences as lost worker productivity and accidents have never been calculated. Moreover, the contribution of sleep disorders to such serious problems as heart disease and stroke, which kill and debilitate thousands each year, has not been quantified.
- Chronic insomniacs reported 2.5 times as many fatigue-related automobile accidents than did non-insomniacs, according to a survey in 1991.
- The same survey documents serious morbidity (relating to disease) associated with untreated sleep complaints, as well as diminished ability to concentrate, memory impairment, failure to accomplish daily tasks, and interpersonal difficulties.

- In the real world, the consequences include learning impairments, discord in interpersonal relationships, errors, and accidents.
- Sleepy individuals are less ambitious and less productive. Sleep loss impairs performance on cognitive tasks involving memory, learning logical reasoning, arithmetic calculations, pattern recognition, complex verbal processing, and decision making.
- The Commission received abundant evidence that insomnia can have devastating effects on the careers and personal lives of those afflicted.
- Individuals who report sleeping six hours or less a night experienced poorer health than those sleeping seven to eight hours per night. Moreover, a nine-year follow-up study found that individuals sleeping fewer than six hours each night had a 70 percent higher mortality rate in comparison to those who slept seven or eight hours a night.
- Forty percent of insomniacs reported the use of either over-the-counter medications or alcohol in an inappropriate attempt to alleviate their sleep problems.
- Patients may engage in self-medication of their sleep disturbances, using alcohol or sedative-hypnotic drugs, leading to further disruption in the sleep-wake cycle and deepening depression.
- For women over the age of forty, the prevalence of insomnia may be 40 percent or higher. Given the data suggesting that insomnia may be prodromal (a precursor) for depression, sleep disturbances could play an important role in mood disorders among older women.
- Twelve million Americans suffer from depression, resulting in annual costs to our society of $10 billion per year. Sleep plays an important role in the onset, course, and treatment of this very prevalent and painful illness.

I found the response to my book from those that knew me very interesting. Even though most were aware of my insomnia, few had any idea of the impact it had on my day to day life. I read that insomniacs somehow muster enough energy to appear to others to be feeling satisfactory. After all, most of us are not hospitalized. There are no cuts or bruises or even bandages or casts to show an outward appearance of trouble. Even though we might have bags under our eyes from lack of sleep, who doesn't? And while some of us complain about not feeling well, others have their problems too. The following statements came from the previously cited Commission report:

- This problem (undiagnosed sleep disorders) is greatly compounded by the absence of public awareness of the profound effects sleep disorders and disturbance(s) may have on the conduct of daily life.
- Perhaps because insomnia is such a pervasive problem, it appears to be accepted as a normal part of life. However, the Commission received abundant evidence that insomnia can have devastating effects on the careers and personal lives of those afflicted.
- The Commission estimates that 95 percent of patients with sleep disorders remain undiagnosed. The cost of these untreated sleep disorders is astronomical in terms of reduced quality of life, lower productivity in school and the workplace, increased morbidity and mortality, and the loss of life due to accidents caused by excessive sleepiness.
- A national survey of 1,105 randomly selected adults reported that, of those who suffered a sleep complaint for seven or more nights each month, 42 percent had never discussed their sleep with a physician.

When the insomniac does discuss his condition with a physician, he is usually his primary care physician. Consider the following findings from the Commission report (Please remember this report was released in 1993 with one of the emphases being to increase education of sleep disorders in the medical community. I have to think there has been improvement since the time of this report.):

- When the family physician does not recognize or lightly dismisses a sleep problem, the patient is not likely to press the matter.
- Despite the fact that insomnia is the most common sleep complaint, few physicians know how to diagnose and treat insomnia appropriately.
- According to a 1991 Gallop Poll, physicians failed to diagnose, or even identify, *one in three adults* who suffers with insomnia.
- A common thread ran throughout the diverse Commission testimony: victims of sleep disorders often described years of frustration, incorrect diagnoses and treatments, multiple referrals to specialists, unnecessary tests, and even institutionalization.
- A national survey of 1,105 randomly selected adults reported that, of those who had seen a physician, nearly three-quarters said their doctor did not ask about their sleep.
- A 1978 study found that fewer than 10 percent of the nation's medical schools provided any education in the area of sleep medicine. A dozen years later, the Commission sponsored a national survey of medical school teaching of sleep and sleep disorders. The study concluded that, while the field has sustained a modest increase in the total number of hours allocated to teaching about sleep and sleep disorders since 1978, a significant number of medical schools still provide little or no time for study in this area.

So, what does all of this information tell us? There are a great number of people with sleep problems costing billions of dollar to this country. Many of these people are trying to treat themselves incorrectly or are seeking advice from a medical community that is ill prepared to help.

Placed throughout the text you will find actual postings I have gathered from Internet discussion groups. Most of the postings came from areas designated for sleep disorders, but a few came from other sites. The authors of the posts are from all over the world. I hope you enjoy the inclusion of these remarks. I had never met or talked with any of the parties when they posted the comments. Their posts do not list names or e-mail addresses unless the author specifically requested the information to be included. The posts have not been edited for the most part. If there has been something edited, it was not for the purpose of changing the intent of the post. I also removed a few words that might be offensive to some readers. The remarks appear as they did on the Internet complete with spelling and grammatical errors. I do not want to imply that the statements are made by experts or that the information in them is true. In most cases there is no way of verifying the qualifications of the author nor the accuracy of the text. Anyone can post a comment, and anyone can respond. The information might be written by a sleep professional or by someone who is relating incorrect information. I find the postings very interesting, much like an electronic version of graffiti.

Introduction

I was becoming pretty excited. I had discovered a way to cure my insomnia. I felt that I could write a book which could help others do the same thing. Knowing that I would really have to struggle with the actual writing, I was nonetheless committed. I knew with my family's help, I could overcome my lack of writing ability. Never mind the grammatical errors, we could correct those. I was more concerned about coming up with coherent sentences that would convey my enthusiasm as well as the actual solution.

My in-laws were in town for the Thanksgiving holidays. Rhonda, my wife, had told them about the miraculous turnaround in my sleep patterns. My father-in-law, never one to mince words, was less than impressed with the idea that I was going to write a book. "What are you going to do, tell them to go to bed and shut their eyes?" After silently thanking him for his constructive criticism, I figured, "What does he know?" He's one of those guys that all of us insomniacs hate, one who say things like, "Well, no, I never have any trouble sleeping. I just lie down and the next thing I know, it's time to get up. Yeah, I go to bed at 10:30 and get up at six every morning. I couldn't sleep late if I wanted. No, I never have anything really bother me when I lie down. Like I said, when it's time to go to sleep, that's what I do."

> *I can remember the first time I had to go to sleep. Mom said, "Steven, time to go to sleep." I said, "But I don't know how." She said, "It's real easy. Just go down to the end of tired and hang a left." So I went down to the end of tired, and just out of curiosity, I hung a right. My mother was there, and she said, "I thought I told you to go to sleep."*-Steven Wright

Well Pop, my father-in-law, may not remember that he also had a fairly severe case of insomnia once when he changed jobs. But, in reality, I should not have thought so badly of him. I am going to try to do exactly what Pop said...help you to go to bed and shut your eyes and go to sleep....all night, without medication. And instead of wondering why he is so lucky to sleep every night, maybe you and I can learn from those that sleep so well rather than asking ourselves, *"Why me?"*

Warning!!

Please be advised that reading the following can and will be extremely habit forming, resulting in nightly recurrences of extreme drowsiness followed by a state of suspended consciousness, better known as sleep. Do not read the following unless you truly want to cure your insomnia and can tolerate the side effects of regular nightly sleep. You have seen all the articles and books and have heard all the things you need to do to sleep better, and, you are convinced, these things just don't work for you. If you seriously want to end your sleepless nights, I want you to take the time to read the following material and follow the easy steps to improve your sleep. If you are starting this with the outlook that there is nothing that can help you, stop right now. Pull it out again when you have yelled at your children just because you are totally fatigued from no sleep. Pull it out because you did not go to work today after getting two hours sleep the night before. Pull it out because you didn't have the energy to go to your little girl's dance recital. Or pull it out because, even though you did everything you were supposed to do and got through the day, it just wasn't any good. Life isn't meant to be like this. The information contained herein absolutely works, but I need your help also. So, if you are ready, settle back and let's take care of your problem. Otherwise, see you in a couple of weeks.

> *Words are, of course, the most powerful drug used by mankind.*
> -Rudyard Kipling

This book will help you with many insomnia problems. You need to consult with your physician to determine whether or not your insomnia has an underlying cause. A breathing problem during the night such as sleep apnea or the use of certain prescription medications are among several factors that can cause sleeping problems. This book is for you if you feel you have ruled out everything else and know that sleeping pills are not the answer.

Part I

THE PROBLEM

You are not alone. You will recognize the story and the symptoms in the following section.

CHAPTER ONE

It's Back
(or Night of the Living Dead...and the Next Day)

It's 3:30 a.m. You can't believe it. This is the third night in a row that you have not been to sleep before 4:00 a.m. You have been in and out of bed all night. When you get up, you watch TV on the couch in the den. Within minutes you find yourself dozing and return to bed only to become wide awake once again. Sleep is so close, and then it eludes you. And the more you worry about it, the harder it is to fall asleep. Your meeting tomorrow is very important and you need to be at your best. There is nothing in your life more disruptive or frustrating. Because of your insomnia, you worry about your mental and physical well-being.

You know somewhere there is an answer, but the answer must lie on some greater level than mortal man can understand. The options are simple. The Lord can either answer your prayers, or you can cut a deal with the devil. If you are praying, please continue. (I know my youngest child used to pray for his daddy to sleep better. My wife used to have her prayer group remember me and my problem.) If you are nearing a deal with the devil, cut off all negotiations at this time. I am about to share the answer that will help you get rid of your insomnia.

You know that later today you will feel wasted, and, as a result, your productivity will be below par. This is not fair to you or your employer. But you have tried everything in the world including sleeping pills. Nothing works. All that you are sure of is that this problem will probably be with you again tonight, or, if not tonight, then the next night. And even if it goes away, it will return after a short respite. You would go to a sleep disorder clinic, but you know there is nothing physically wrong with you, and you do not want prescribed sleeping medication or to be referred to a psychologist for evaluation. Aren't the people with mental problems the ones who go to psychologists? There is nothing mentally wrong with you. Besides you have neither the time nor the money to go. Therapy probably wouldn't work anyway.

It is now 4:00 p.m. Somehow you made it through the day. You were so exhausted you were unable to do any productive work, but you did make it to the meeting. You should not get fired, at least not for failing to attend the meeting. Never mind the fact that you were so tired you neglected to finish the proposal that was due today for your most important client. Never mind the fact that your insomnia-induced fatigue, demonstrated in your job performance, is preventing you from being promoted. Today was about survival only. If you can just sleep well tonight, you will get back on track at work tomorrow....hopefully.

Earlier, at lunch today, you fought the urge to go home and take a nap. With a nap you might have been able to be more functional during the afternoon, but you knew better. A nap just would have made things worse. Tonight you and your spouse have been invited by some friends to go out to dinner and a movie. Both of you have been looking forward to this. You dread calling your spouse and telling her once again that you are too tired to go out. All you want to do is go home and crash. You are going to have to cancel the racquetball match with your friends after work also. You always have fun with them, but not today. *Life is supposed to be better than this. Much better.*

It is now 10:00 p.m. When you first arrived home, you were so sleepy that you thought about taking a nap again. You could have been asleep in two seconds. But you have been there and done that. You knew if you took a nap, your sleep tonight would be worse than the last several nights. As usual, dinner did somewhat revive you. Between 7:30 p.m. and 10:00 p.m., although you were still worn out, you felt more alert than you had all day. You had some interaction with your family, but mainly you were tired and irritable. You also realize that, when you feel this tired, you seem to eat more than normal. It's as though your willpower has been suppressed along with the rest of your energy supply, so you end up compounding your overall problems by eating too much. You are physically and mentally exhausted and know that it is critical that you get a good night's sleep. As bedtime approaches you become more anxious knowing you will probably end up tossing and turning once again, repeating the same ritual from hell that you have faced most nights recently. *How can you be so tired and still unable to sleep? You need help and you need it right now. There has got to be an answer.*

11:00 p.m. You know the drill. As tired as you feel, you are becoming certain that tonight will be no different from the last several. You decide to try to lie down hoping that you are wrong and will find sleep tonight. As a matter of fact, you feel yourself getting really sleepy after laying your head on the pillow. You are almost there. Then POW! You are wide awake again. Exhausted, but wide awake. Perhaps you even dozed off for a minute or two. But the cycle continues. *You cannot continue to live like this. "What is the answer?"*

Subject: NEED SLEEP!
From: issamk@julian.uwo.ca (Issam Kobrsi)
Date: Tue, Feb 10, 1998 10:21 EST
Message-id: *

I NEED SLEEP!!!!!
In the past 4 months I'm averaging less than 10 hours of sleep
a week. It is really disturbing me!!! All night laying in bed
all I can think of is getting to sleep but my eyes don't even
shut for a second! I't getting me frustrated and during the
day I'm a walking time bomb ready to snap at someone,

anyone! I am missing most of my morning classes because
of this. when I finally fall asleep at 6:30 there's no way in
hell I'm getting up by 7:30!
HELP!! what should I do?? sleeping pills? I'll do anything
to get a good night sleep.

Awake until 4am
Posted by * on December 13, 1997 at 23:48:34:

Hi all,

I don't know if I am in the right place- but it was recomended
that I come talk to you. I am awake until 4am or 5am every
night these days and since I have to be up for work at 8am
this is causing a lot of problems. I have tried cutting out
caffee, excersizing more (albeit half heartedly) and staying
up all night to see if I just need to break the cycle. Nothing is
helping me much. Does this sound familiar to anyone? Any
advice or thoughts?

i am so tired I feel like I have the flu all the time. Any help
would be appreciated. (Oh yeah, I have been given Xanex
which helps but then I can't get out of bed to go to work. A
real problem too....)

CHAPTER TWO

My Credentials

Let me introduce myself. My name is John Wiedman. I am a mortgage broker with a degree in finance from the University of Memphis. I am forty-eight years old. I live in Memphis, TN. I do not have a Ph.D. specializing in clinical psychology from some big name university. I have not been in charge of a center for sleep disturbances for the last fifteen years. I am, however, a professional insomniac (or at least I was until recently). I have had regular bouts of chronic insomnia for more than ten years and sleep problems for much longer than that. I can help you rid yourself of insomnia. And although I am not much of a writer, I will try to present this information as effectively as possible. I am writing this from the perspective of an insomniac. I have found the answer to my insomnia, and I will do my best to convey to you the steps you need to take to treat yours.

I am not attempting to circumvent your relationship with the medical community. This book is for those of you that have already talked with your doctor, and nothing short of sleeping pills will provide even temporary relief. My assistance is directed at those of you that have fallen into regular routines of insomnia and need to learn the solution to your problem. I think this book should also help those of you that have recently developed insomnia by showing you how to prevent your problem from becoming more chronic.

If you have not already told your doctor about your sleeping problem, you need to do so. As I stated earlier, your insomnia may be caused by some other reason such as an existing medication or sleep apnea, and he may be able to help. Have him help you rule out any obvious reasons for your insomnia. If you feel you are currently addicted to a sleep medication, work with your doctor to wean yourself off the medicine. Tell your doctor you are going to read this book. If he is skeptical about any of its contents, have him read the book. It is not very long. *I would appreciate it if you have him buy his own copy. I need all the sales I can get.* Otherwise, use this book. It will provide you with the tools to help treat your insomnia without any medication or herbs or alcohol.

While your initial insomnia may have been caused by any number of reasons, now your insomnia is more than likely a habit you have formed that is comparable to biting your fingernails. And, unless you are currently taking a sleep medication and have formed an addiction, eliminating insomnia from your life is going to be easier than quitting tobacco or any other addictive substance. But while biting your fingernails may be an annoying habit resulting in unattractive nails, insomnia can wreck the quality of your life. There will be no unpleasant withdrawal symptoms like there are when you quit smoking. Everything that results will be positive. *In my case, I slept much better from the first night, with only one really bad night in the first thirty. I cannot begin to tell you how absolutely remarkable that was.* I had just come out of a cycle where, for three nights out of five, I was awake until four or five o'clock in the morning. At most I may have dozed sporadically before the time I finally went to sleep. The next day I would be absolutely worn out, unable to concentrate for any significant period of time. Needless to say, my irritability was a real pleasure for my family. I was upset. *Why me?* I knew there were many others who had sleeping problems like me, but why were we singled out to suffer?   And not only was I too tired to work efficiently, I was lucky to get any work done at all. The only thing that kept me going was pure adrenaline. When I slept this poorly, I found it almost impossible to muster the energy to exercise, further compounding the overall problem. Additionally, I was canceling out of social functions with my wife, children, and friends, again due to my fatigue. In other words, any semblance of a normal lifestyle was gone. And the good nights weren't much better, but at least I sometimes got four or five hours of sleep. I may have awakened several times, but the quantity was better.

Being a professional insomniac, you can rest assured that I have experienced almost everything that you have...the worry, the frustration, the anger, the prayers, the endless late night infomercials (whatever happened to the hair in a spray can?). I know every psychic or promote-a-psychic from Kenny Kingston to Dionne Warwick to Sylvester Stallone's mother to the guy with the white brillo pad on his head...if you have seen him, you know who I mean. I have also been enticed by all shapes, sizes, and colors of women from around the world willing to share their most intimate secrets. Want any information regarding abdominal machines, juice machines, or losing weight? I'm the man to see. I know whom to see to make a fortune in direct marketing or real estate. I never did see the one middle-of-the-night infomercial that I thought was a natural: how to cure insomnia. After all, who do they think is watching in the middle of the night?

I know what it is like to toss and turn and get in and out of bed all night watching the clock go slowly from midnight to 5:00 a.m. *Why me?* As I lay in bed for hours, my mind would race with thoughts about the employee I must discipline tomorrow, or I would get madder over something one of my children had or had not done. I have lain in bed for hours with seemingly nothing occupying my thoughts, still not falling asleep. I have gotten up and watched television all night. I have gotten up and read all night. I have gotten up and worked or straightened my office or played on the computer, you name it. I have drifted off to sleep only to awaken within minutes and not go back to sleep. I have slept for a couple of hours only to awaken and never get back to sleep again. And I have done it night after night after night. Trust me, I have gone through just about anything that you have, maybe worse.

And, is it just me, or has anyone else ever noticed that it is harder to sleep when there is a full moon?

---

full moon
Posted by * on April 11, 1998 at 23:47:35:

anyone else have trouble sleeping on nights when there is a full moon?

I have tried sleeping pills, antidepressants for sleeping purposes, melatonin, warm milk, exercise in the late afternoon, exercise in the morning, exercise in the evening, sleep clinics, over-the-counter medications (including aspirin, Advil, Benadryl, Nyquil), hot baths, a glass of wine, one or more stiff drinks, "white noise", soft music, TV on, total darkness, night lights, and both the presence and absence of a clock in the bedroom. I have stopped smoking, don't drink coffee, have gone to caffeine-free drinks, and don't take afternoon naps. My wife and I went from a queen size bed to a king size with a firmer mattress. I have used a heating pad and tried sleeping in different positions. If I could not fall asleep, I would get out of bed rather than staying there tossing and turning. Nothing stopped my insomnia-until now.

Re: insomnia, melatonin

Posted by * on October 09, 1997 at 12:41:19:

In Reply to: Re: insomnia, melatonin posted by on October 05, 1997 at 20:59:21:

I have a friend that has tried everything: melatonin, warm milk, sleeping pills, leaving the room after sleeplessness, etc. Lately he has been taking sleeping pills out of desperation.

He says his stress level is normal.

Subject: Re:Insomnia{Sleepless in Boston}
From: (Rac)
Date: 1997/03/19
Message-ID: *

hi All:
Yesterday, I purchased a bottle of Valerian Root capsules. I took 4 last night{475mg each}, per suggestion of clerk, no sleep! Does this Root take time to get into one's system, or does it simply not work for me? Is the "herb" route for some, and not for others? Melatonin does nothing for me either. Any advice on overcoming insomnia woukd be greatly appreciated, especially since it's been going on for years! I've done the sleep labs, clinics, Drs. ect!

Thanks in advance!!
Ron

Depending on my frustration level at any particular time, I would pull out my books and read everything I could get my hands on regarding insomnia. I have symptoms of several classifications of insomnia, caused by several types of stimuli. I have trouble falling asleep as well as staying asleep. My mind races, my mind doesn't race. I have stress, anxiety, and depression (Who wouldn't, with no restful sleep?). I have restless legs syndrome (RLS), periodic leg movements (leg myoclonus-PLMS), night eating disorder, conditioned insomnia, Sunday-night insomnia, my circadian rhythms are screwed up, and now, as I am growing older, I am being told my sleep is not going to be as restful as it was when I was younger. WELL, THAT'S JUST GREAT!!! And don't even get me started right now on sleeping medications or the sleep clinic that costs hundreds of dollars. The doctors at the sleep clinic prescribed a medication for anxiety saying that I was a type A personality. Thanks, but no thanks!

Insomnia is a gross feeder. It will nourish itself on any kind of thinking including thinking about not thinking.-Clifton Fadiman

CHAPTER THREE

I Did It, So Can You

There was one thing that I always thought about during those many wasted hours. I was going to figure out a way to beat the monster. I would lie there and be so tired and so close to going to sleep, and the monster would grab me again just as I was dozing off. *Why me? What have I done to deserve this?* Insomnia has literally cost me hundreds of thousands of dollars. Because of my sleeping problems, I left a very good job to work out of my home so that I would not be tied to a schedule. I have done satisfactorily, but nothing like I was doing before. Since that time I have been presented with several opportunities for employment that no normal person would ever have rejected. "Yes, I will be happy to start on Monday. By the way, occasionally I have nights (about 3-4 a week) where I don't sleep very well, and I don't function quite as efficiently as you might like me to. Don't worry though, if I don't get to sleep by 5:00 a.m., I have a rule that I just call in sick". Because of my insomnia, I wouldn't even schedule a haircut appointment until 10:30 in the morning. If I had to attend an early morning meeting the next day (before 10:00), I slept even worse worrying about getting up on time. And how great did I feel when my wife told my son that Dad would not be coming to his early morning soccer game because he did not sleep well last night? Again, all of this has now changed.

> *When you come to the end of your rope, tie a knot and hang on.*
> -Franklin D. Roosevelt

I always told myself that when I did figure out a way to beat my insomnia, I would take my knowledge and help others. When I was awake at three in the morning, absolutely exhausted, with sleep nowhere in sight, I used to look for something that would just push me over the top....sleep was so close, yet so far. There had to be a way. Well, glory, glory, hallelujah! The day has come. I want to share with you the peace of mind that I have found. Don't let anyone tell you that you will never sleep normally again because I am living proof that you can. Don't let anyone tell you because of your age that you will never have a good night's sleep without a sleeping aid because you can.

Let me tell you about my sleep last night. First of all, I have now been "cured" for seven weeks, and it keeps getting better. Last night I went to bed at midnight, ready for sleep. Before my "cure", I would have been dreading the time when I finally had to lie in bed and attempt to go to sleep. Last night I had to struggle just to make it to bedtime. I fell asleep almost immediately. I woke up once, thought about getting up, decided not to, and slept the remainder of the night until 7:00 a.m. Can I hear an "amen"? Can you even remember what a night like that is like? I cannot honestly remember a night like that in over ten years, unless I had taken a sleeping pill. Then I felt somewhat hung over the next day. Compared to my sleep in the preceding months, I have had only three marginally bad nights in the last seven weeks. My bad nights now are comparable to or better than my best nights before. Many nights I go to sleep within minutes and only wake up two or three times. I may get out of bed once or twice. Again, last night I never got out of bed and only woke up once, resulting in a refreshing seven hours of sleep.

Why should you listen to a mortgage broker with a degree in finance? Your doctor has not been able to help you other than to give some general advice and maybe prescribe a sleeping pill as a short term solution. Why should you listen to me when you know someone that has gone to a sleep clinic staffed by sleep specialists and still has a problem sleeping? Why should you come to me when there are stacks of books and articles on the subject of insomnia written by sleep experts with better credentials than I have? Well, as I told you, I am a professional insomniac. I have the advantage of on-the-job training as well as having read many articles and books on sleep disorders over the last few years.

Before my "cure", I had reached a point where I had started skimming recent articles for some new breakthrough that might help me, instead of reading the complete story. Most of the information was usually a retread of something I had read before. There are many good tips and suggestions that come from those books and articles, which I have incorporated into the cure that worked for me. There are also many suggestions that, in my opinion, are superficial. To me, the tips on sleeping better are somewhat analogous to all the tips I used to get on my golf game. To correct my problems in golf, I would think about how to grip the club, the correct backswing, how to hold my head, keeping my left arm straight, the proper follow-through, and on and on and on. No wonder I never hit the ball well! There were too many thoughts going through my head. A good golfer does not have twenty thoughts going through his head as he addresses and strikes the ball. His body moves naturally and freely, resulting in a ball well struck. Sure, he makes minor corrections from time to time, but his mind is not breaking down each segment of his swing on each stroke. Likewise, a good sleeper should probably do exactly what my father-in-law said. A good sleeper goes to bed on time, shuts his eyes, goes to sleep, and wakes up the next morning feeling refreshed. I am going to help you make a few minor adjustments in your sleep routine so that you can also achieve natural free-flowing sleep.

You probably have read some of these same articles and books. You have seen the special reports on television that tease you with help for insomnia but never deliver. Is there good information in the articles you have read or in the reports you have seen on television? Of course there is. But they really didn't help your problem with insomnia, did they? Most of what I will tell you came from a combination of my personal experiences as well as personal research.   But the end result was only achieved through trial and error. I am going to present the information to you in such a way that you will see the steps necessary to treat your insomnia...without drugs, without a costly visit to the sleep clinic, and without going to a psychologist. I will present the information and the solution to you from someone who really understands what you are going through and show you how to overcome the little problems along the way.

Change your thoughts and you change your world.-Norman Vincent Peale

Part II

MY EXPERIENCE

This section really serves two purposes. First, it is a form of my personal sleep biography which you can use as an example in preparing your sleep biography. Maybe it will help you to look a little harder at those events which shaped your current sleep habits. Secondly, it is a description of my sleep related experiences, such as taking sleep aids, in terms you might have read in other books or articles on insomnia. I will also show how various sleep disturbances affected me. Hopefully, it will help you in understanding your current condition. Most of you will see yourself in many of the situations I describe when you read this section.

CHAPTER FOUR

History

From The Start

When I was young, I believe I slept pretty well. I do know that I talked and walked in my sleep quite a bit. I can remember spending the night at someone else's house on several occasions and waking up in another room. I got banged up several times while trying to get back to my bed in the dark. I could never figure out how I could see to get around in the dark while sleepwalking but could not see a thing once I awakened. I would stumble into furniture and trip over objects on the floor. Also, I awakened on several occasions in the street in front of my house. If I recall correctly, I was dreaming someone had entered my house while I was there alone, and I escaped to the street so as not to be trapped inside with the intruder. And like most children, I did my share of talking in my sleep. While these facts may not qualify me as a childhood insomniac, I think they show clearly that I was not on the straight path to a perfect night's sleep later in life. For the most part I grew out of sleepwalking and talking by my early teens.

In retrospect, I believe many of my bad habits that led to my later career as a professional insomniac began in high school. In elementary school I can remember waking early enough each morning to eat breakfast and read the paper before going to school. But in high school, I began to stay up later and later, sleeping until the last possible minute the next morning with no time to even eat breakfast, much less read a newspaper. This left me just enough time to arrive before the late bell rang at school. I still don't think that I had a problem with getting to sleep or staying asleep, though getting out of bed was getting harder and harder. Then, in the summer of my junior year, I had a job where I did not have to report for work until 3:00 p.m. I can remember sleeping later and later all summer until I was actually sleeping until 2:00 p.m. As a result I was staying awake until four and five in the morning. Obviously, once I drifted into this pattern, I had difficulty adjusting to normal hours once school began again.

In college I continued my high school routine of staying awake too late and then sleeping until the last possible minute the next morning. Certain aspects of college actually made the situation worse. Whereas in high school, when classes started at the same time every day, the classes in college were available with a choice of class times. During my freshman year, I actually took Tuesday and Thursday classes that began at 6:30 a.m. and ended at 9:30 a.m. I thought this would be a great idea because then I would have the rest of the day to study, work, or play. Instead I would come home and nap for a few hours. In subsequent semesters, I began to schedule my first class as late as 1:00 p.m. on certain days, thus allowing me to sleep very late.

Period Napping Vs. Full Night Sleep

Posted by * on February 12, 1998 at 18:11:13:

As a college student, I find it very difficult to maintain a regular sleeping pattern. One night I pull an all nighter, the next day I nap for hours. Often times, I am not tired untill 4 or 5am. After months of trying to force myself to go to bed at a descent hour to be refreshed for the following day, I have had enough. Ideally, I would like to take 2or3 3-4hour naps a

day. Is this healthy? Would I feel refreshed and be able to
carry through with my daily routines? Thanks.

The first time I can really recall having trouble falling asleep
was when I was in the National Guard. I would have weekend
duty where I had to report by 6:30 a.m. Still in college, my earli-
est classes were never before 9:00 a.m., and getting to the Guard
by 6:30 a.m. was somewhat of a challenge. On Friday and Saturday nights before weekend drills, I can remember tossing and turning in bed, knowing that if I didn't get to sleep soon, I would not
be very effective the next day. I can remember on several occasions going to bed much earlier than usual in an effort to get
plenty of sleep, but that just made matters worse. This was the
first time in my life that I remember feeling totally fatigued the
next day as a result of insomnia.

Other than those problems I encountered while in the National
Guard, the first real problems occurred on those occasions when
something really had me keyed up at work. I was working in
mortgage originations, and the volume of work was so heavy that I
worked ten to twelve hour days just to keep my head above water.
Every minute was high energy, and I would come home
exhausted. I worked very hard and was constantly keyed up. I
kept getting promoted until I had quite a few people working for
me. Logically, there would be occasional employee problems.
When I had an employee problem, I would begin to wake up in the
middle of the night and worry or get mad. I finally made a rule for
myself that when I began to lose sleep over a problem, I would
face it head-on the next day. I felt this tactic would keep the problem from causing any additional sleepless nights. Unfortunately,
knowing that I now had to confront the employee in a somewhat
uncomfortable meeting the next day would further keep me
awake. And to compound matters, I was usually worn out from no
sleep when the meeting actually took place. Personal problems,
such as a problem with one of my children, would have the same
effect on me, a racing mind resulting in tossing and turning all

night. Even those events that I looked forward to would keep me awake. I loved a new snowfall and would stay awake all night watching for the predicted snow to fall, just like a little child. I coached youth basketball and would lie awake thinking about the big game coming up. Those restless nights were generally temporary in nature, only lasting a night or two. Then I would return to my normal routine of "satisfactory" sleep. However, a very negative pattern was starting to develop with regards to my sleep. The occasional bad nights were becoming more frequent.

---

only have insomnia when i really don't need it

Posted by sasha on April 08, 1998 at 05:29:19:
s.l.stephens@sussex.ac.uk

My problem is that normally I can sleep fine; normally, that is, when there is nothing going on in my life which is exciting or important. However, if I ever have something to look forward to, for example, Christmas, a party, a holiday or even a night out I simply will not get ANY sleep the night before which makes it impossible to enjoy the event. As soon as I hear the news of something fun or exciting I start to get stressed at the very thought of the sleep I know I am going to miss. I know this is a self fulfilling prophesy but I have tried telling myself not to worry about it. I have tried sleeping tablets . Please can someone help, I feel that I am condemned to never enjoy myself again as the sleep problem stops any planning for the future.

Any advice greatly appreciated

sasha

About fifteen years ago my situation really started to deteriorate. Not all at once, but night by night matters just seemed to get worse. Previously, I had occasional bad nights when I was awake a good portion of the night.   Now the bad nights were coming more often.   I don't intend to go into every detail of my decline, but I will say the change for the worse coincided with a couple of job changes.   The first change was from a high energy office environment to working out of my house as a field sales representative.   Although I continued my past pattern of hard work, I was not under the same constraints as I had been while working in a corporate office.   I would occasionally sleep in when I had stayed out late entertaining customers or after one of my occasional sleepless nights.   While it initially felt good to go back to sleep, I usually felt groggy for the rest of the day once I finally got out of bed.   You know the feeling after you have stayed in bed too long.   In retrospect I don't think my body really wanted or needed the extra sleep, and it only served to adversely affect my sleep the next night.

My next job change found me back in an office. My new job allowed more freedom from time demands than my previous jobs. When I first came to the job, I was astonished by how much free time the other salesmen seemed to have.   Also, most of the salesmen would leave right at the scheduled quitting time, if not before.   I had always worked hard with ten or more hour workdays.   The new job, while not easy, was basically cold calling (trying to sell a product or service to someone I had never talked with) on the telephone.   It was not unusual to stop several times a day to chitchat with others to break the stress of constant rejection on the phone. My previous jobs had required me to work very hard just to keep up with the workload.   Once I had established a few good accounts in my new job, I could work them for only a few hours each day and still make good money.   The rest of the time could be spent working or goofing off.   I truly think this had an important impact on the development of my subsequent sleep habits.

Sleep Clinic

From that point on, whether or not the amount of work was the actual determinant, my sleep habits worsened. In February of 1990, after complaining to my doctor regarding my sleep habits, I was sent to a new sleep clinic that had opened in a local hospital. I was guardedly optimistic. With all due respect to you with sleep apnea, I was hoping there would be some physical reason for my inability to fall asleep. Then they would tell me what I needed to do to correct the problem, and I would sleep happily ever after. But I was afraid the outcome would just be a verification that people with my type personality have problems sleeping.

My experience at the sleep clinic was not very positive. Before going to bed, the clinician put a cord with a clip on my ear and another on my nose, connected electrodes all over my body, and routed them to a belt that looked like a carpenter's or electrician's belt. Then from the belt came a main cable that ran to wherever the recorders were located. I had to grab the main cable and give it a tug every time I needed to move in bed. If I wanted to go to the bathroom, I had to signal the attendant to come and disconnect the wiring. I was very surprised I was allowed to eat a snack after I had lain down. I had developed a habit of craving food both late in the evening and after lying down, which contributed to my sleep problems. Needless to say, I did not sleep very well that night. *After reading this section my son, Brad, suggested we call them "no-way-to-sleep clinics".*

The second night was better only because I was totally exhausted from the night before.

Can't sleep during sleep studies !

Posted by * on November 18, 1997 at 13:14:15:

I just returned from my 2nd sleep study. Both times I had difficulty going to sleep. The 1st night I slept 1-2 hours, the 2nd night I was able to sleep about 3-4 hours. I'm not sure

why I couldn't sleep, but it's very frustrating. Is this a
common occurance? Any suggestions?

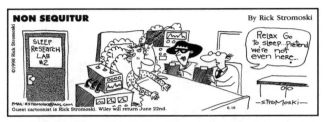

© 1998, Washington Post Writers Group. Reprinted with permission.

From my "sleep disorders evaluation" for the nights of February 27, and February 28, 1990, the following was reported. On the
first night I was awake two hours and forty-four minutes of the
seven hours and forty-two minutes in bed (which was more sleep
than I actually thought I got). The clinic further reported that it
took me thirty minutes to fall asleep. Once asleep I had 172
arousals of less than thirty seconds and 16 awakenings of more
than thirty seconds. Out of the 172 arousals, 120 were attributed
to leg myoclonus. From the books I have read, leg myoclonus
(commonly referred to as periodic limb movements in sleep or
PLMS) is described as a leg condition in which a person's legs
move uncontrollably for a few seconds while the person is sleeping (there is a subsequent chapter dealing with this subject). I am
very familiar with this as my wife had this condition several times
about a year ago. While I would be lying in bed, trying to sleep,
her legs would start moving every twenty to thirty seconds. I
would find myself starting to count the time between the movements (for all of you that always ask what an insomniac does all
night, here is one pathetic example). Her leg movements would
come in intervals almost to the exact second. She would never
wake up or consciously be aware of the episodes. She would admit the next day, however, to maybe being a little more keyed up
than normal before going to sleep, or she might have exercised

late that night. I would occasionally place my leg over hers to see what would happen, but she would still try to move her legs right on cue. If I held my leg over hers for any period of time, she would ultimately shift away.

Leg jerks and RLS
Posted by * on September 24, 1997 at 22:28:49:
I have had "busy" legs for as long as I can remember, but it was never more than that. Over the past two years though, I have developed (and it's getting worse) some strangeness that I have come to know (through Internet research) as RLS and PLMS. The symptoms I have experienced have caused me relationship problems, discomfort and embarrassment.

It started out as simple discomfort in the legs (while I was awake) which caused me to cognitively keep my legs moving in some type of motion. My wife then started making comments about how restless I was when I was asleep. It stayed this way for about a half year. Then things got worse.

Every evening when I started to relax I found my legs twitching, this was not uncomfortable but it was embarrassing (my family felt I was doing it purposely). It was not long thereafter that my wife started accusing me of having sexually based dreams in which I was acting out the "act" while I was asleep. When my wife would wake me, I had no memory of dreams......

Today, my twitching has turned into "jerking", and it happens any time at any place where I find myself relaxing/shutting down. The jerks are powerful enough that they will knock my Pomeranian off of my lap. I've also had the jerks while driving and standing. My restlessness in bed has been better controlled through regulation of caffeine and sleeping on my back, but it's still a problem (the caffeine levels don't seem to affect the jerking much).

My concern primarily relates to the jerking, because it seems to be getting worse. What do we know about the process that brings on the jerking. Is it related to brain activity? How is it related to the restlessness that I'm experiencing in my legs and the body movements I experience while I'm asleep?

I would appreciate any help.

So, the leg myoclonus, which this clinic referred to as "periodic movement of sleep", was listed as the first cause of the "disorder of initiating and maintaining sleep". The second cause listed was generalized anxiety. This conclusion was derived from a psychiatric survey given to me. I guess the fact that I reported I had a "hyper" personality and worked extremely hard probably helped them reach this conclusion also. They informed me that my type of personality usually had the most trouble sleeping well. As I told you, I had always refused to take any medication for sleeping except for the one time. Based on the clinic's finding, I was given a prescription that would help, not only to put me to sleep, but to slow me down in general. This, in turn, would help me sleep. When I grilled the doctors about the drug, I was assured that it was not addictive. They did admit I might have some problems sleeping if I happened to run out of the pills or leave them at home when I went out of town. They said I should take the pill every night for a "prolonged period of time", although not for the rest of my life as "no medication is prescribed for the balance of a lifetime".

---

wake up after 2 hours cant fall asleep again

Posted by * on September 26, 1997 at 17:41:18:

am 74 yrs Male..went sleep clinic 8 yrs ago. All they could do was prescribe more drugs with side effects.Have tried seconal,halcion,dalmane,restoril and just attempted ambian 5mg..got side effects of dizziness. Others became addictive.Whats left ??I cant stand it..I am on vasotec and

mevacor-aspirin . Had a by-pass 12 yrs ago. Dont drink
coffee except decalf and only for lunch. Dont smoke. Retired
and no debts or worries. Please help!!

They also said I should benefit from behavior modification but felt that the drug should alleviate my sleep problem. This clinic did not offer behavior modification training or support as part of its services. They sent me back to the physician who had referred me to the sleep clinic, and nothing ever came of using behavior modification. Knowing what I know today, even if I had pursued the behavioral solution, I would have had difficulty finding someone with the proper training to help me.

Furthermore, the technicians could not understand why I complained about the belt and cable, which I felt negatively impacted my sleep while at the clinic. They told me most people in the clinic did not have a problem with the wiring. I say if those people could sleep with all that equipment, they probably didn't need to be there in the first place. I have to think the method they used on me was technology in the early stages...sort of the Model T of the sleep monitoring profession.

When I went to the pharmacist to get my prescription filled, I was told that the drug prescribed for me was Klonopin, a drug used primarily to treat seizures but also used to treat anxiety and as a sleeping aid. He said it could be habit forming, contrary to my doctor's assurances otherwise. Although the initial dosage was not very high, it was to increase after a couple of weeks according to the prescription. As a result, I never got the prescription filled.

Subject: For RLS/PLMS, Klonopin didn't work - What next?
From: *
Date: 1996/12/12
Message-ID: *

I was recently diagnosed with PLMS (periodic limb movement syndrome) in addition to my obstructive sleep apnea. I had an average of 2 legs movements per minute during the sleep study.

The Doctor put me Klonopin to help control the PLMS, but unfortunately I found that I was getting a few undesriable side effects. Mainly, I became much more irritable and impatient during the day, I felt even more tired and less rested than before the medication, and I completely lost my sex drive. Because of this, the Doctor told me to stop taking the drug to see if the symptoms went away - which gladly they did.

I go back to see the Doctor next week, and I would appreciate hearing from other people with RLS or PLMS. I'd like to know if you've had similar problems with Klonopin, and what medications or treatment finally worked on you.

I do not mean all of this as an indictment of sleep clinics. I told everyone from the onset that I was not going to start taking medications (thanks for the advice, Mom), much less one that could be habit forming. I think the clinic I went to was wonderful for some people, particularly those with sleep apnea. Unfortunately, I was not one of the lucky ones. Since the time that I was at the clinic in 1990, I have read about certain treatments, such as light therapy, as well as counseling for depression and anxiety, that were not mentioned or tried with me. I can only assume these alternative treatments were not covered by insurance or actively practiced at that particular time.

Subject: Question about Sleep Disorder Clinics
From: *
Date: 1996/03/11
Message-ID: *

I know all sleep disorder clinics are different, but I was
wondering if they generally only deal with sleep aphnea (sp?)
(as my doctor said) - or if they also deal with my problem
which is getting to sleep in the first place. I have had this
problem since mid-October, so far the only "plan of attack"
has been various medications, which work most of the time
but are not solving the problem.

I recently phoned a local sleep clinic to check things out, as it
had been seven years since my visit. Their particular program be-
gins with personality testing and drug screening in order to uncover the factors that are causing the patient's insomnia. Also, a
one night's stay is usually recommended so that the patient's sleep
pattern can be monitored. The personality testing and drug
screening cost about $250 with the overnight stay costing about
$1500 more. Depending on the doctor's recommendations, the
patient may also have additional tests the following day. If behavior modification is suggested, the patient is referred to a second
clinic in the hospital run by a local university.

I also phoned the same sleep clinic where I had stayed almost
eight years ago. Posing as a prospective patient, I asked for the
doctor and was told by the receptionist that she could probably answer all of my general questions. I asked her what would happen
if an evaluation basically found me to have poor sleep habits and
recommended behavior therapy for my problem. She told me that
they did not have an in-house program dealing with behavior
modification (she also said they did not do any work with light
therapy), but that they could give me a pamphlet on sleep hygiene.

Insomnia and sleep clinics

Posted by * on December 12, 1997 at 16:46:46:

I have been coping with chronic insomnia for 14 years now, averaging about 5 hrs sleep a night, if I'm lucky. Docs have not been much help. I have quit using caffiene and alcohol, practice stress reduction and meditation techniques and am managing the condition as best I can with 1/2 mg doses of klonopin, but I don't consider that a cure. I have been looking for a favorable referral to any sleep clinic. The Stanford Clinic seems to be the most famous, yet the 2 people I spoke to who were treated there 10 years ago could not give it a favorable word. I had a full evaluation 5 ½ years ago at the Northwest Sleep/Wake Disorders Program-no diagnosis came from it. Has anyone suffering from long term chronic insomnia had a successful treatment at any clinic or with any doctor? By successful, I mean that one leaves with a physical diagnosis leading to some treatment which ends with the subject able to look forward to 8 hrs of unmedicated sleep a night.
Any replies please email *

Sleep Cycles

My sleep tends to run in cycles. The bad cycles were characterized by little or no sleep until four or five in the morning. I am cognizant of the fact that sleep studies show that most people actually get more sleep than they think. There have been nights when I would lie down and get up five or ten minutes later thinking that I had never been asleep. My wife would tell me later that for a few minutes I was dead to the world and, seemingly, out for the night, only to get up almost immediately and be wide awake. t is not uncommon for anyone waking from the first stage of sleep to be unaware of being asleep. Insomniacs apparently have more problems than others recognizing they have been asleep in the early stages of sleep. This can cause additional frustration for the insomniac. What I do know is that, even if I had been asleep, it was for only a few minutes. During the remainder of the time, until five in the morning, I had been on the couch wide awake either reading or watching television. Then, when I finally did lie down, I would sleep lightly for a couple of hours.

Even when I was in a relatively good cycle, things were actually pretty bad. In a good cycle, I would try to go to bed around 11:00 p.m. to midnight. I would usually get back up within fifteen to thirty minutes and return to the den. I would then stay up until I felt I was ready for sleep, typically somewhere between 2:00 a.m. and 3:30 a.m.. Even after falling asleep, I would get up several more times, normally for a short duration. Then I would usually get out of bed around 8:30 a.m., though it could be later depending on how much sleep I actually got and how rested I felt.

A great night for me, which would occur maybe one or two days a month, would be to fall asleep around midnight and to awaken and get out of bed only four or five times. The next day I would feel wonderful. When I did have nights like these, they were almost always followed by a really bad night. It was almost like I was being punished for getting a good night' sleep.

Self-Employment - Probably a Mistake

Later that year I left my job to work out of my house. I was having more and more problems sleeping, and my company would not tolerate tardiness. On the nights when I got very little sleep, I was like a zombie the next day at work, just going through the motions. I thought that if I only got a few extra hours of sleep by working out of my home, I could function somewhat better, so I made the change. At home, if I did not get to sleep until very late, I could at least sleep to 8:30 or 9:00 the next morning. Instead of helping my sleep problem, the horrible cycles came more often and lasted longer.

I have found in talking with others that many insomniacs are not on a structured work schedule; that is not to say they do not have a full day's work to perform, but they have some flexibility. Self employed persons, housewives (sorry, domestic engineers), students, consultants, contract laborers, and retirees among others tend to have the kind of schedules that permit some flexibility. Unfortunately, we insomniacs have a tendency to use this schedule many times to try to catch up on lost sleep by sleeping late or taking daytime naps.

CHAPTER FIVE

Sleeping Disorders

Night Eating Syndrome

For some time my sleep problems were being further compounded by what is called "night eating disorder" (or syndrome), a condition where there is little hunger or eating during the morning followed by bouts of bingeing after dinner with the onset of sleepiness. My appetite was almost insatiable. So the more tired I became, the more I snacked, usually eating sweets or high fat snacks. And guess what? The more I ate, the more impossible it became to sleep properly. Talk about something to look forward to as bedtime approached each night! Additionally, I would get up and eat all night, waking me up even more (can you say, sugar buzz?). Not only did I not sleep, I gained a couple of pounds, or so it seemed, each night. Also, when I ate late at night, my legs became very restless. I will discuss that problem more a little later.

So here I would be on the couch about 10:30 p.m., sort of dozing. Against my better judgment, I would eat a couple of cookies. Then I would go back and eat more. Before I knew it, the whole package was gone, though I really was not that hungry. Suddenly I was more awake than I had been all day. Then to top it off, my legs would become so restless, I felt like I would scream. Time to sleep? I don't think so. Then after I finally did go to sleep, I would awaken and eat snacks all night long. When I would awaken the next morning, I would have little or no appetite, beginning the cycle all over again.

When I read books and articles about sleep disorders, I am always amazed that there is not more information about night eating syndrome. As a matter of fact, the doctor at the sleep disorder clinic in 1990 noted that I related a desire to eat sweets when I awoke during the night. The only comment the doctor made about the condition in my report was that I had gained weight as a result the late night eating. I did find one article in USA Today, a few references on the Internet, and a brief mention in a book. The articles all describe the condition exactly, indicating it is an eating disorder, but never suggesting a cure. I have read theories that the disorder is due to emotional problems, stress, a hormonal imbalance, low blood sugar and/or food addiction. I am afraid that it is just another malady caused by a myriad of reasons. About the only thing that most sleep disorder books and articles suggest is that you do not eat heavy meals or snacks late in the evening, particularly those that are spicy, those that have caffeine (including chocolate), or those that are high in fat or high in sugar. Most sleep experts will tell you not go to bed either with a full stomach or feeling hungry. Most don't even mention this night eating disorder. I know mine is triggered when I become more sleepy. I don't know if there is a psychological explanation for the disorder, but I do know that it is extremely disruptive to normal sleep habits. Many insomniacs have told me they have the same problem. They were somewhat comforted to find out others had the same condition.

I have also noticed that my appetite is usually greater on those days when I am more fatigued than normal due a lack of sleep the night before. On those days, I tend to crave food during the daytime also. Some of the factors I have read that contribute to increased appetites include depression, boredom, and anxiety, all of which are worse on days following little or no sleep. I have read that limited human studies have linked sleep deprivation to an increase in appetite.

eating throughout the night

Posted by * on October 03, 1997 at 18:30:49:

I have been suffering from night eating for years. I wake up
several!times a night and eat food. It doesn't matter what it is.
I am fully awake. I will be sleeping very soundly and wake
up suddenly and make my way to the kitchen. I've tried
everything! Locking myself in my room, eating three good
meals a day, not buying food etc. I've often thought of
hypnosis. I'm not even sure if it's a sleep problem or an
eating problem, but why can't I sleep through the night
without getting up for food. I'm not necessarily hungry when
I do this. I don't know.

Subject: Re: Night eating
From: *
Date: Sat, Mar 7, 1998 17:43 EST

I have been doing the same thing for over 10 years now, and
have yet to find a solution. Like your friend, I almost always
wake up 1 hour after getting to sleep,and feel an
uncontrollable urge to eat. Sometimes I wake up 1 time a
night, other times up to 4 or 5 times a night, and it never has
anything to do with how much or little I've eaten during the
day-I eat whether I'm full or not. I do suspect the waking part
has to do with a screwed up circadian rythm, and how much I
eat has to do with the amount of stress I'm feeling. though
I've somewhat made peace with this habit/disorder, I am still
looking for solutions. I have been to sleep specialists, who
have put me on meds (prozac, and various other
antidepressants) but nothing works. I recently have been trying high doses of melatonin (up to 20 mg, with time
release) but that doesn't seem to work either. Tell your friend
he can e-mail me privately if he wants (he can use another
name) since I've never met anyone else with this problem,
though I know others do have it. my e-mail is: *. It would
be interesting to compare notes and feelings.

Before I start feeling too sorry for myself, there is another sleep disorder that is called sleep eating disorder. Victims of this disorder not only eat after they have been in bed but also while they are sleep walking. While I was at least awake when I had one of my middle of the night binges, these poor sufferers are not even aware of what is going on during the episode until they get up the next morning and find the evidence. Like those with night eating syndrome, they also tend to eat large quantities of food that are usually high in sugar or fat. The victims have been known to eat food that is raw, frozen, and spoiled. The menu for the night has included salt and sugar sandwiches and even buttered cigarettes. Obviously their trips to the kitchen can be dangerous in addition to being unhealthy from an overeating perspective.

Restless Legs Syndrome

Restless legs syndrome, known in the medical community as RLS, is a condition where there is an irresistible urge to move one's legs when sitting or lying down. My legs become extremely restless. I feel like I have demons in my legs, and I need an exorcist to cast them from my body. It is impossible to sit still without being uncomfortable. This usually occurs when I get very tired in the evening prior to going to sleep, although it can occur during the day if there are periods of inactivity such as driving a long distance or watching a movie.

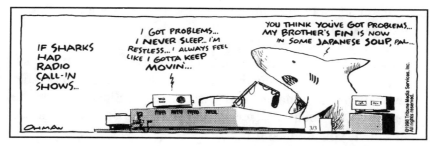

© Tribune Media Services, Inc. All Rights Reserved. Reprinted with permission.

Most of the time I don't do anything to alleviate the discomfort other than stretch or walk around. I have found that sometimes the best relief is to focus my attention elsewhere until the unpleasant sensation leaves, sort of a Lamaze-type solution. My wife swears that taking a long, very hot bath eliminates her problem. Since the initial draft of this book, I have finally listened to my wife for a change and found that her solution of taking a hot bath works better for me than anything else I have ever tried. Without fail, I get some degree of, if not total, relief. The following is a list of other recommendations that I have heard or read that are effective at certain times for certain people. It would be worth a try to see if any of these alternatives can provide you with enough relief to avoid medications and their side effects.

- Take very cold baths (as opposed to very hot baths mentioned above)
- Get regular exercise
- Stretch the muscles and ligaments in the back of your legs from the calf muscle to the area behind the knee
- Sit in a chair so that the edge of the chair does not hit the back of the legs
- Use a heating pad
- Use cold packs
- Massage the affected area
- Take aspirin or ibuprofen
- Take vitamins and other supplements where there might be deficiencies. (See your doctor for any vitamin and supplement recommendations that might be appropriate in your particular circumstance).
- Wear long socks or stockings
- Avoid all forms of caffeine including coffee, tea, soft drinks, chocolate, certain medications (Pay particular attention to diet medications, stimulants, and certain pain relievers...Ask the pharmacist for help in determining if your medication contains caffeine if you are unsure)

Also, since the initial draft of this book, I have found a book devoted to restless legs syndrome called <u>Sleep Thief</u> written by Virginia N. Wilson. Ms. Wilson is an eighty-three year old who has suffered with restless legs all of her life. In addition to relating her own experiences, Ms. Wilson, who is not a medical professional, is joined by fifteen RLS specialists in the book. The book made me realize that my symptoms are not nearly as severe as many of the victims mentioned in the book. The book points out that RLS is now being diagnosed in young children who previously were thought to have "growing pains". The book further points out studies that show RLS to be hereditary. From my perspective of trying to avoid medication if at all possible, I felt as though there was too much attention to the pharmaceutical treatments and not enough for alternative treatments. It is pointed out that while certain alternative treatments (such as those above) have shown to be effective for some, others derive no benefit from the treatments. As a result, the alternative treatments can't be recommended by the Restless Legs Syndrome Foundation. On the other hand, much is made of the medications used to treat the disorder with the acknowledgment that the disease and related symptoms usually never go away completely. The problems of tolerance, rebound symptoms, and associated side effects of the medications are discussed, however.

Ms. Wilson was also a cofounder of the Restless Legs Syndrome Foundation, a nonprofit agency that supports research, provides information about RLS, helps develop support groups, and publishes a newsletter, *Night Walkers*. The Foundation has a site on the Internet with an address of http://www.rls.org/ that provides a wealth of information regarding the disorder. The Foundation also makes available a free information bulletin about RLS and the Foundation that can be obtained by sending a stamped (55 cents postage as of June, 1998), self-addressed envelope (business size #10) to :

Restless Legs Syndrome Foundation
PO Box 7050
Department JW
Rochester, MN 55903-7050

As I told you earlier with my "night eating disorder", I grow hungrier as I become sleepier. If I ultimately give in and eat, my legs will often become very restless shortly thereafter. While this condition does not occur every night, it is usually much worse when I eat late in the evening on a night when I am very fatigued.

On a final note, most people that have restless leg syndrome also have periodic limb movements known as PLMS. If you recall, this was the main diagnosis I received as a result of my visit to the sleep clinic. A sign of PLMS is usually seeing bed sheets that are in total disarray upon awakening in the morning. Also, your spouse may complain about you kicking or thrashing about during the night. As far as I know, I no longer demonstrate any symptoms of PLMS. Is my PLMS gone without medication?

---

actual affect of meds in RLS

Posted by * on January 20, 1998 at 04:26:27:

Hi guys, Im new here. Im recently dx'ed with RLS and taking 1mg of klonopin. What I would like to know is, are the medications supposed to stop the leg movements, or just help you sleep better? At first, I found I was sleeping all night, but all the sheets were still at the bottom of the bed. Now I dont seem to get any benefit at all, except that I get to sleep easier. Which never really was a problem. My problem is staying asleep. I saw a sleep Psychologist who made the dx, then turned me over to my m.d. How do they measure effectiveness? more sleep studies? That was my worst night sleep ever. Please respond by email, as I dont get here to often.

thnx
*

In Reply to: Re: restless legs posted by * on November 22, 1997 at 20:17:29:

At last there is a name for my crazy legs. I feel like I have electical currents in my legs and can't keep from moving them i the middle of the night -also when I have to sit still at the theatre - I am the one squirming around. Benadryl worked for 2 nights, I've tried Soma (perscription), potassium glotomate - but not much helps. I would love info and suggestions.
*

Circadian Rhythms Disorders

Our sleep is regulated by internal body clocks known as circadian rhythms which means "about a day" in Latin. Unfortunately while the rest of the world is on a twenty-four hour clock, our internal body clock may be different, with many people having a twenty-five hour body clock. Our job is to continuously work to coordinate this body clock with the real world. Exposure to sunlight is a key component to keeping your circadian rhythm on schedule. Thus people who work night shifts or who are not exposed to much outside light are more apt to have problems. Typically indoor lighting is not a viable substitute for exposure to sunlight. The control of body temperature is a key function of circadian rhythms. Our bodies are more alert during high temperature periods and more ready for sleep during our low temperature times.

Not everyone's internal body clock is set the same. Some people have a short circadian rhythm resulting in the person falling asleep earlier in the evening and waking earlier in the morning. This is called advanced sleep phase syndrome. Other people have a longer circadian rhythm, go to sleep later, and sleep later in the morning. Their condition is called delayed sleep phase syndrome. Both of these conditions are sometimes being treated successfully with light therapy (discussed below). In addition, delayed sleep phase syndrome can be treated with the plan that I describe later in the book.

Has anyone heard of this sleep disorder?

Posted by * on November 19, 1997 at 03:41:54:

My sleep problem is as follows:

I don't know if this is a sleep disorder or not. Perhaps it is a symptom of another problem.

My average sleep time length is between 9 to 11 hours, my average waking time is 15-17 hours.

As you can see, the extremes cause a natural "rotating schedule" .That is, if I fall asleep at 10pm on Monday, wake at 8am on Tuesday, I will not be able to fall asleep until at LEAST 11pm on Tuesday night, and the shift continues. If I try to wake up to "correct" the cycle, I feel extremly tired and it lasts most of the day.

Any suggestions? I've seen my PCP about this. His diagnosis left me un-satisfied (i.e. "Just get to bed sooner") . Was considering going to a sleep disorder clinic, but dont have thousands laying around just for them to tell me that.

*

There is another sleeping problem linked to circadian rhythms in the winter months due to the shorter number of hours of light each day. The condition is referred to as seasonal affective disorder or SAD. The problem is compounded by the fact that there is a tendency to stay indoors more during that time of year.

Symptoms include the inability to fall asleep, fragmented sleep, difficulty in getting out of the bed, energy loss, craving sweets and starches, depression, and weight gain. The disorder appears to become increasingly worse when the number of hours of daylight decreases. *In addition to all the parties we all go to in the winter months, could this be another factor in our seasonal weight gain?* One of the methods being used to treat this disorder is light therapy, also called phototherapy. In this treatment you are exposed to bright light early in the morning, a process which helps to reset your circadian rhythms to normal. I read an article in my local paper that reported that coffeehouses in Stockholm and Helsinki now offer light fixtures that simulate sunlight. The sun only shines about six hours a day in these locales and even then struggles to shine through thick gray clouds. Patrons report being happy about the addition to the cafes.

Although I am not aware of specifically having this disorder, I seem to have more difficulty sleeping in winter months. I guess I thought that was due to being more inactive in the winter. For more information on this disorder, go to the Web site for the Society for Light Treatment at http://www.websciences.org/sltbr/ or you can write to them at:

SLTBR
10200 West 44th Street, Suite 304
Wheat Ridge, CO 80033-2840

I am aware of some companies that sell the fixtures. You can get information both on the disorder and the intended impact of the lighting by contacting them. I am sorry if there are others that I am omitting.

Apollo Light Systems
352 West 1060 South
Orem, Utah 84058
800-545-9667

The SunBox Company
19217 Orbit Drive
Gaithersburg, MD 20879-4149
800-548-3968

Subject: Re: What is SAD?
From: "monique paré" *
Date: 1998/02/19
Message-ID: *

Hello *,
I have SAD and phototherapy has been wondeful for me. In addition to phototherapy, I try to do exercise every day and go outdoor when it is possible. If you have Internet, this is a good place to have information on SAD. If you don't have Internet, email me and I will send you more information.

Many peoples, specially in autumn and in winter, when days are shorter and light is less intense than in spring and summer feel depressed, tired, want to be alone,etc...Others symptoms : excessive sleeping and eating, weight gain, loss of libido. It could be a kind of sickness named SAD - (seasonnal affective disorder.)

Seasonnal affective disorder (SAD) is a disease caused by the lack of light and is very well known by psychiatrists and doctors. It is treated by phototherapy, (bright light therapy). A very good book, well-documented on SAD is "Winter Blues" of Dr Norman Rosenthal. He says that having more knowledges on the symptoms of depression is the beginning of recovery
Good luck,
Monique.

Conditioned Insomnia
(Learned Insomnia)

Conditioned insomnia is like the granddaddy of all insomnias. According to the books and articles I have read, conditioned insomnia occurs when you are able to fall asleep just about anywhere other than your own bed. Regardless of what originally caused your insomnia, you now associate restless nights and insomnia with your bed and bedroom. If you are on the couch or in a hotel room and have no problem sleeping, you probably have conditioned insomnia. So here is the deal: Whatever caused the initial bouts of insomnia may no longer be a factor in disrupting your current sleep habits. However, the act of getting into your own bed now consciously or unconsciously triggers some kind of response recalling the restless nights you have been experiencing and interferes with falling and/or staying asleep. *You are lying on the couch. You find yourself dozing, unable to remain awake. You retire to your bedroom convinced you will fall asleep. You lie down in your bed. Just as you think you are about to drift off, you are suddenly wide awake again.* Obviously, this is a problem. This is one of the reasons you are encouraged to get out of bed when you have trouble sleeping. You do not want to associate your tossing, turning, and general anxiety about falling asleep with your bedroom. I have no doubt that conditioned insomnia was one of the major factors in my progression to becoming a professional insomniac. I will reference this subject again in the following solution.

Conditioned insomnia

Posted by * on February 10, 1998 at
13:45:41:

I've suffered with conditioned insomnia for five years, have visited two sleep centers (one for an overnight study which found nothing), eight different professionals (psychologists, psychiatrists, counselors, hypnotists, etc.), and have tried every anti-depressant, anti-anxiety medication known to man. Results? Not! The most sleep I ever get is 5 hours, and I'm a walking zombie all day. I've driven through red lights, stop signs, hit the gas when I should have hit the brakes, etc. I've screwed up royally at work, and my income as a result has dropped precipitously. I need help. I mean, I really, really need help. I'm certain what I have is conditioned insomnia, for a number of reasons, but I don't want to bore you with all the details and background here.

Please, can anyone walk me through the steps of getting out of this hellish sleeplessness? I am desperate.

I will do anything! Thanks.

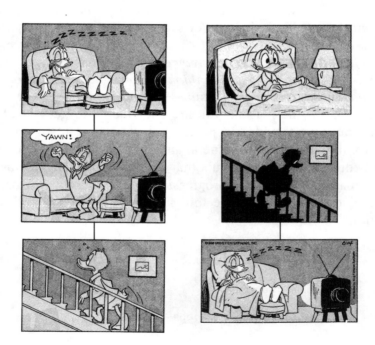

© Disney Enterprises, Inc.

Sleep Apnea

From the National Commission on Sleep Disorders Research report referred to in "A Note to Readers", it was reported that, "Sleep apnea alone is the cause of excessive daytime sleepiness experienced by almost 20 million Americans". I do not have sleep apnea, at least I didn't when I last visited my local sleep clinic. Sleep apnea and insomnia are different classes of sleep disorders. And although this book is about insomnia, anyone who has insomnia must rule out sleep apnea as a cause of his sleeping problems. Also, many victims of sleep apnea also suffer from insomnia.

There are several types of apnea. Obstructive sleep apnea is characterized by the intermittent discontinuation of breathing during sleep due to the obstruction and/or collapse of the throat. Central Sleep Apnea is a neurological condition causing the intermittent cessation of breathing during sleep. Mixed apnea combines the two aforementioned apneas.

Symptoms include snoring, awakenings caused by gasping for breath, and excessive daytime fatigue. You may not even realize that you have these symptoms unless there is someone in the bedroom who complains about your snoring, gasping, or thrashing around in your sleep. Your daytime drowsiness may have become worse without your realizing what has happened. *Until you were diagnosed as nearsighted and fitted with new glasses, you didn't know your vision had deteriorated, did you?* Having one or more of these symptoms does not mean you necessarily have sleep apnea. The only way apnea can be diagnosed for sure is by staying overnight in a sleep clinic. In a later chapter on sleep clinics you will be advised how to find an accredited sleep clinic.

Just like those of us with insomnia, those with sleep apnea, diagnosed or not, are searching for an answer to their dilemma. Many of the medications and herbs used to combat insomnia can be even more dangerous for use by those with sleep apnea by making breathing even more labored than it currently is. Likewise, alcohol can relax the airways creating more problems. If you have any of the symptoms of sleep apnea, it is even more important for you to look at the techniques touted in this book before taking any sleeping aids. And do go to a sleep specialist for an evaluation.

Subject: Insomnia and Apnea
From: *
Date: 1997/12/12
Message-ID:*

First of all, thanks to the people on this group, who helped me understand what sleep apnea was a couple of years ago. I have not posted here before, but have frequently read the messages.

Since late 1995, I have been using CPAP. It has changed my life. It has given me alertness and energy I never thought I'd have. That is, until recently.

A couple of weeks ago, I started waking up at 3AM, and unable to go back to sleep. This seems different from the OSA, in that I wasn't waking up repeatedly.. just once. My nasal pillows were still in place, and I couldn't go back to sleep.

Then around the middle of last week, I stopped falling asleep. Some nights there was no sleep, sometimes 1-3 hours, but never anywhere near the 8 I usually get. I've missed four days of work because of extreme fatigue.

I have been on Halcion since before the apnea was diagnosed, and also take Melatonin. Plus Prozac and a bunch of meds unrelated to the sleep problem. My doctor isn't sure whether to refer me to a Phychiatrist or Neurologist, because we're not sure what's wrong.

Do the experts here think this is an apnea problem, or some other kind?

Treatments for apnea include surgery, weight loss, dental appliances, and the use of airway pressure devices known as CPAP and BPAP. These devices blow air into your nose keeping your air passage open. The long term effects of untreated sleep apnea can be very harmful.

I do not know the accuracy of the information below. I do know there is considerable information relating to the medical consequences of sleep deprivation over a long period of time.

Subject: Sleep Apnea and your chances of being 60
From" *
Date: Tue, Jan 20, 1998 07:22 EST
Message-id *

Hi all,

I read in a recent US medical output that SEVERE sleep apnea is rare amongst people over 55, not common amongst people 50-55 and very common among people below 50 and above 30 where the same group of people are people prone to having sleep apnea. The survey concluded that the reason that it was rare to find SEVERE sleep apnea sufferers over 55 is because of something they termed "The SURVIVOR Syndrome" which bascially meant that most people dont live beyond 50 and very few past 55, who have SEVERE Sleep Apnea (you people with mild are not included in this). The reason it thinks this is the case is basically the strain on the heart, as we all know.

I would like to hear what people think of that. I am seeing a heart specialist again tomorrow, for the first time since 1993. I know, personally, that I get worse every year not better. What about the rest of you?......................................

An excellent Internet site for information on sleep apnea is, http://www.newtechpub.com/phantom/faq/osa_faq.html. Also the American Sleep Apnea Association, which was founded to promote education and awareness of apnea can be reached at:

> The American Sleep Apnea Association
> 1424 K Street NW, Suite 302
> Washington, DC 20005
> Phone: 202/293-3650 Fax: 202/293-3656
> Web site: http://www.sleepapnea.org.

There is also a book often recommended about sleep apnea that I have not read, with one author being a medical doctor and the other a sleep apnea victim, called <u>Phantom of the Night: Overcome Sleep Apnea & Snoring</u> by T.S. Johnson M.D. & Jerry Halberstadt.

There are a couple of very good Internet discussion groups listed in the "Support" chapter later in the book that deal extensively with sleep apnea. There is also a sizable section in the Internet listing in the Appendix of this book concerning the subject.

CHAPTER SIX

Sleep Aids

My First Sleeping Pill

In spite of all the problems that I had over the years, I had always said I would never take a sleeping pill. I really can't remember the exact reason I have always been so reluctant. Maybe my mother, who was a registered nurse, convinced me of the perils. I know I had heard horror stories of people who had to take pills to go to sleep, then more pills to get going in the daytime. The ultimate outcome was almost always tragic. I made a decision that I would suffer the consequences of insomnia rather than turning over control of my life to a bottle of pills. I never had a problem with taking an antibiotic that would fight infection or an antacid that would take care of my heartburn. My concern was with those drugs that affected mood or personality or habits with questionable results and potentially dangerous side effects.

In any event, when my doctor set up my appointment at the sleep clinic, he asked me to try one Halcion before going to the clinic to see how I reacted. He had hoped a couple of sleeping pills might be the thing to get me back on schedule. I reluctantly agreed. If you know anything about Halcion, it was the drug of choice during this period. Halcion was different from other sleeping pills in that it knocked you out like a sledgehammer. In any event I took one and did not fall asleep until 5:00 the next morning.   So much for the sledgehammer effect.   Somehow I knew my body might react like that.

Over-The-Counter-Medications

Based on what others told me about their various degrees of success with over-the-counter medications, I have tried just about everything at one point or another.   My problem was that most of the over-the-counter medications did not have the desired effect on me.   They actually seemed to wire me up and keep me awake rather than gently lulling me into the elusive dream world.   While others said Nyquil did the trick, I lay awake.   Sominex, the same. Excedrin PM, ditto.   If it put others to sleep, it woke me up.   I had people swear by Benadryl.   I became keyed up when I took it.

In Reply to: natural remedies posted by * on October 08, 1997 at 22:15:03:

Have you tried over-the-counter remedies like Tylenol-PM? It's not what I would call natural but sure has worked for me. The secret ingredient (PM) is diphenhydramine HCl, an antihistamine (Benadryl). Has worked better than anything else to help me go to sleep and stay asleep for 7-8 hours. Only problem is you build up tolerance to it after awhile. I also don't know if there are side-effects associated with long-term use. BUT, for short-term use...try it! I would prefer using a more natural approach, but none of those worked for me.

I have tried melatonin, and it seemed to help for a while.   After adjusting my dosage several times, I quit taking it.   I just didn't see a benefit any more.   Out of desperation I finally decided to try an occasional sleeping pill and initially began taking Restoril (te-mazepam).   I only took one on rare occasions.   If I were in a cycle where I was up until four or five for several straight days, I would take one to try to get back on schedule. The pill would sometimes help me get a good night's sleep, but I usually would not be able to sleep very well the next night. It was as if the sleep gods would not let me have two restful nights in a row. The occasional pill would, however, give me a day that I could feel somewhat better and sometimes might even help me break out of the bad cycle for a short time. The only other time I would take a sleeping pill was if I knew there was an early morning meeting or appointment that I was required to attend. Although the pill would allow me to get some sleep, I still had to overcome the grogginess which made concentration hard the next day.

---

prescription for sleep?

Posted by * on December 03, 1997 at 10:22:53:

What prescription medications are best for sleep problems? I've tried all of the OTC stuff like Benadryl, melatonin as well as a glass of gin. I've tried them all with poor results. I keep to a regular schedule, avoid caffene and try to do "all the right things". My family doctor doesn't consider sleep disorders a "real" problem worth treating. I have a close friend who is an MD, and he is willing to help....but sleep is not his specialty. Any suggestions on a pill that will put me to sleep and is relatively safe?

I have read various articles that question the dosage of melatonin that is most often taken. Melatonin is typically sold in dosages of two to three milligrams. Some researchers feel that anything more than 0.3 mg is too much, so the dosages being sold are significantly too high. High dosages of melatonin have resulted in insomnia in some users. High levels of melatonin have resulted in side effects the following day, such as problems with alertness.

The use of melatonin as a sleeping aid has been effective for many, while others derive no benefit or experience only short term results. Most of the success seems to occur with shift workers who are able to use melatonin to reset their body clocks. Likewise, those traveling across time zones, such as airline pilots, have had varying degrees of success resetting their body clocks. No study that I am aware of has established the effect of long-term use of melatonin, and for that reason, caution must be exercised. If you take melatonin regularly, you should keep your physician aware of your use, be on the lookout for any unusual symptoms, and continuously watch for any new studies that might help you determine the safety of your choice.

The use of vitamins, minerals, and other supplements should be monitored by a qualified professional. There is a misconception that your body will discharge unused amounts of these substances without any harm to you. Indiscriminate use of such products has led to toxic levels of the substance in the user. I have read that excessive doses of some vitamins have resulted in dependency. Certainly, I am not against the use of vitamins and other supplements; I am just saying use them wisely and consult a qualified professional if you have any questions. Too much of a good thing may be harmful. Deficiencies in magnesium, zinc, copper, iron, and calcium as well as some of the B vitamins can impact sleep and should be monitored on an individual basis.

Benzodiazepines

In the seventies, a new class of sleeping pills replaced barbiturates, which had been used prior to that time to treat insomnia. If you recall, Marilyn Monroe died of an overdose of barbiturates. Barbiturates are rarely used to treat insomnia today. The new sleeping pills, benzodiazepines (BZDs), include triazolam (Halcion), which I mentioned earlier, and tamazepam (Restoril) among others. Another BZD is clonazepam (Klonopin), which is generally prescribed for the treatment of panic disorder but is also used to control the symptoms of restless legs syndrome and periodic movement of limbs in sleep, both of which I have already discussed.

Other than the one Halcion that I had tried, my first real introduction to BZDs came after my sleep pattern continued to worsen. Someone told me that he had heard of "cycling" sleeping pills. He explained that I should take the pills for a week or so to get back into a normal rhythm and then discontinue the usage before becoming addicted. He found this to be the way that sleeping pills worked best. I had reached a point of desperation but still was sure I would not use sleeping pills other than for a short trial. I called my doctor, who was not in, and explained my request to his nurse. She agreed that "cycling" the pills could be effective and said his office would phone in a new prescription for temazepam. She said not to worry as the temazepan was not that strong anyway, that they had patients who had taken it every night for years without a problem. I was pretty psyched up about "cycling" the drug. The first night I slept well and felt pretty good the next day, especially with the promise of six more days and nights like this to follow. I did feel a little hung over, but with the extra sleep, I still felt much better than normal during the day. The second night I slept well again, and the next morning I awoke feeling pretty good. By mid to late afternoon, I began to feel even more of a hangover which lasted the rest of the day. The third night I slept, but not as well. The next morning I woke up feeling even more hung over. By mid afternoon I started feeling a little wild. By late afternoon I felt like the men in white coats were coming to get me. I felt exactly the way I did when I quit smoking after twenty years. I had problems concentrating and became very irritable. My kids didn't know what was happening, but they learned quickly to stay away from me. My wife said the look in my eyes and my coloring were the same as when I had stopped smoking. I stopped the "cycling" of the sleeping pills after feeling the way I did on the third day. When I met with my doctor later and told him what had happened, he told me I should not have listened to his nurse, as she did not know as much as she thought she did. I had naturally assumed that he was aware of her advice to me and the fact that she had phoned in the prescription. Ultimately, I did go back to taking pills, but only as a last resort during a really bad cycle of not sleeping well. I took no more than one pill a week.

All that was achieved by taking a pill was to get an occasional good night's sleep. Then I would go back to the same routine on the other nights when I didn't take medication.

You will note that I started having powerful side effects from the medication after only three days. I have heard and read mixed opinions as to whether or not an addiction can be formed in three days. Some firmly believe you can become addicted that quickly if you have an "addictive personality". Others say that you cannot become addicted that quickly. They say you might be having some sort of withdrawal, but it does not necessarily mean there is an addiction. All I know is that my body and mind were telling me, in spite of a more restful night's sleep, to quit. And they weren't telling me quietly. They wanted to make sure I understood the point by making the side effects worse than the fatigue from staying awake all night.

Subject: Help! I'm addicted to Restoril!
From: *
Date: 1997/12/18
Message-ID: *

I'm a 27 year old female law student. I have a history of severe insomnia. When I get an insomniatic period, I don't sleep at all for days. This last time I went 72 hours without any sleep and the doctor perscriped Restoril (Temazepam) - a benzodiazapine.
Usually I have a strict rule that I only take drugs on the second night of my insomnia to "break the cycle," but the doctor told me to take them every night and get on a regular sleep schedule. I'm on one now, and trying to cut down the dosage of medicine, but its not working. Does anyone have any similar experiences of 1) the type of insomnia where you can go for days and days without sleep? (I once went for 5 days, but that was before I discovered drugs.) and 2) how to get off this xxxx?
Basically, my big fear is that if I just stop taking them, I won't sleep for days. I don't know why my body doesn't eventually just get sick and fall asleep, but it doesn't .Help! -

---

Subject: GAD and insomnia...
From: *
Date: 1997/02/20
Message-ID: *

Tried Klonopin yesterday, .25 in the moring, .25 at night, felt like a zombie. Stick to the .5 ativan during the day and it's "jittery feeling" until I can find something else. At least I can function. The nights haven't been to good. Still waking up after a couple of hours on ambien. Gonna try restoril. Take care...

Ambien - The Next Generation of Sleeping Pills

Last year I began hearing more and more about a new sleeping medication called Ambien that supposedly had none or few of the negatives of benzodiazepines and other sleeping aids. The generic name for Ambien is zolpidem tartrate, and it is a member of the imidazopyridine class. I had been told by one doctor friend that the medication was either available without a prescription in Europe or in the process of being approved for over-the-counter use. The indication was that it might be a safe alternative. I was going to a new doctor at this time and he agreed that, because of the severity of my insomnia, I should try Ambien. When I went to the pharmacy to pick up the medication, I asked the pharmacist what her experience had been regarding the side effects of Ambien, primarily the addictive potential. She told me that any time she has "little old ladies" (I use that term affectionately) come across the counter when told their personal doctor would not approve another refill, the medication in question is probably addictive. This sounded logical to me. She also suggested that I ask my doctor regarding the use of trazodone, an antidepressant she said many doctors recommend because it aids the sleep process without addiction and subsequent withdrawals. That night I called about fifteen different pharmacies and got the same answer from all but two...Ambien is potentially addictive, take trazodone instead.

I called my doctor the next day and inquired about the use of trazodone. He suggested before taking trazodone that I take one 10 mg Ambien nightly since I had not even tried one yet. I experienced the same problem that I did with Restoril, by the third day feeling as though I was losing my mind. My doctor then suggested I cut the dosage in half or try to cut back to every other day. He was not a big advocate of trazodone saying we would explore other alternatives if cutting back on the Ambien did not help with my side effects. Even with the milder dosage, I had the same symptoms of feeling half crazed and extremely irritable by late afternoon with the men in white coats standing by. I knew I would never take sleeping pills again, other than maybe once a week at the most.

Subject: sleeping pills
From: *
Date: Wed, Jan 28, 1998 09:35 EST
Message-id: *

Anyone have trouble with sleeping pills? I started taking
them (my husband's prescription) because i was sleeping
poorly, then kept with them to stop me from going
downstairs to eat late at night (helped somewhat, but don't
do it) and now I seem "addicted " Can't sleep without them.
Ambien-only taking ½, but tried to cut down to ¼ and
couldn't sleep.

Subject: Re: ambien w insomnia
From: *
Date: Mon, Feb 23, 1998 16:04 EST
Message-id: *

I can't get to sleep until close to daylight. Should I have an early appointment I just stay up.

My doctor prescribed Ambien and said to immediately go to bed for it would take effect within ten minutes. It didn't put me to sleep. After about a week I found myself getting very dizzy whenever I stood still. I stopped taking Ambien and in a day or so was OK. Another trip to the doctor where she told me to take it every three days. That didn't help me sleep, so I stopped taking them. At the next visit she put me on valium. Doesn't help me get to sleep but I'm not as cranky and my wife likes me better.

Trazodone

At this point I was ready to try trazodone, but I knew my new doctor probably wasn't going to go for the idea. In addition to not wanting to prescribe an antidepressant for me, he was worried about some of the side effects. I looked through some paperwork from my former doctor, whom I no longer trusted as a result of the problem with his nurse. In the paperwork, I found an old prescription for trazodone which I was able to get filled. The pharmacist was shocked as the prescription called for me to take 300 mg at bedtime. The normal starting dosage for sleep related problems is in the 25-50 mg range. The 300 mg was a dangerous starting dosage (you see why I did not have much confidence in the first doctor), so I only started out at the 50 mg level. I will have to say this, trazodone was everything the pharmacists had told me. I did not go to sleep nearly as quickly as I would with a sleeping pill. However, once I fell asleep, I stayed asleep and woke up without any hangover feeling. More importantly, at the end of the day, I did not develop the nervous withdrawal-like feelings. I took the trazodone continuously for a month and a half. I might have had nights where I did not go to sleep until 2 or 2:30, but then I slept well for the remainder of the night and awoke feeling fresh. Probably the biggest initial negative side effect that I experienced after taking the dosage of trazodone for the evening was the extremely uncomfortable bouts with restless legs syndrome. Additionally, when taking trazodone and then eating, it was like turning up the volume on the RLS by 300%. Once I fell asleep, I got a good night's rest while taking trazodone, but the symptoms from the restless legs many nights were almost unbearable and would cause me to remain awake until one or two in the morning. This did not happen every night, and the degree of discomfort was almost always directly related to how much I ate after taking the trazodone. Even without eating, there usually was some discomfort, but not always.

The other side effects were for the most part as advertised. On the negative side, my mouth was dry, although this was never much of a problem. In fact, the dryness was no longer noticeable after several days. Additionally, I experienced a reduced sex drive. I was not particularly pleased about this side effect, but I was willing to sacrifice to a degree in order to sleep better again.

I definitely felt more rested during the days following trazodone usage, but there was some feeling that life had slowed a little. My wife was really impressed that my temperament had improved so dramatically. I believe my improved temperament was due to the fact that I was so much better rested, not so much to any antidepressant effect of the drug. In any event, I must have been a little more laid back. I noticed that I lost some of my aggressiveness, but that was a satisfactory trade off. I was sleeping much better. Never mind that my concentration was not quite as good as before (on a well-rested pre-trazodone day anyway). Without sleep my concentration had not been quite as good anyway. On the positive side, my resting heart beat, which had recently been very high, now had dropped significantly. Even while sitting on the couch, my heart beat had been in the 90-100 range. After using trazodone, a heart rate in the 60's and 70's was common. Prior to the use of trazodone, I had borderline high blood pressure with an average of about 135/88, with higher readings depending on the severity of my insomnia. After trazodone my blood pressure would be 115/70.

I did have a few questions I needed answering. I knew I could not go to my former doctor who gave me the trazodone prescription as I was no longer a patient. My new doctor didn't know I was taking the trazodone. I got most of my questions answered by pharmacists. I still wanted to know if I should take trazodone nightly for the best results. About once a week my wife and I have a glass or two of wine, and I knew antidepressants and alcohol were not the best of mixers. Also, I had increased my dosage to 75 mg a night and once again felt the beneficial effects were beginning to diminish. I wanted to know if I were going to continuously have to increase my dosage due to tolerance to the drug. I noticed the stronger the dosage, the worse my concentration became. The pharmacists kept telling me to ask my doctor. Finally, I called the staff pharmacist at the drug manufacturer who was there to answer inquiries like mine. All the staff pharmacist said was that trazodone was not intended for the treatment of insomnia and refused to answer my questions. Somehow, I don't think the company objected to anyone buying its product for that use. It just disavowed any knowledge of its use as a sleep aid. The company's pharmacist finally humored me by saying that the dosage I was taking should not create any adverse problems for me.

I eventually stopped taking trazodone when I was up to the 75-100 mg level a night and was still having trouble sleeping most nights. Additionally, my concentration became so bad on some occasions that I could not read two sentences in a row (if I did, I certainly could not comprehend what I had read). I also started having problems with simple math calculations. Even my wife, who had really enjoyed my more mellow personality, realized what was happening perhaps was not worth the benefits. Obviously, once I stopped taking the trazodone, the chronic insomnia returned. I tried on various occasions to start out with a 50 mg dosage once again, but never regained my initial success without increasing the dosage with the resulting problems.

Subject: Experiences w/ trazodone??
From: *
Date: 1997/02/10
Message-ID: *

Hi everyone. I am new to this newsgroup though not new to
sleep problems; have long had sleep disturbance connected
w/ a long-term illness. I'm wondering if anyone has
personal experiences/info to share re: using trazodone to
sleep. I'm having a helluva time starting on it —even at 25
mg/night I wake up a few hours after falling asleep w/
intense heart palpitations & nausea w/ trouble getting back
to sleep. I take it w/ a little bit of protein/carb food so I'm
confused as to these reactions. Maybe I am hypersensitive to
the drug & should try something else? Does anyone have any
tips to offer?

Thanks!!

*
*

In Reply to: Re: Trazodone posted by * on October 04,
1997 at 19:18:16:

I too have been prescribed Trazodone for Insomnia. I have
experienced nightmares, and daytime sluggishness and
headaches. I believe the cure is even worse than the
symptoms. I am in the process of looking for more natural
remedies. i've not had luck with melatonin but hear Valerian
root works. I plan to try it and will report back.

Subject: Re: Experiences w/ trazodone??
From: *
Date: 1997/02/11
Message-ID: *

Hi *, I'm new to this group, too. I was on Trazadone to help me sleep, but all it did was stuff up my nose to the point where I couldn't breath. I couldn't tolerate it at all. My doc switched me to Ambien, which only worked for a few days. Now I'm on Amitriptyline, which thankfully is working. You might want to check this out. (Has anyone else used these drugs?)
Good luck!
*

Alcohol

It always amazes me how many people use and recommend alcohol as a sleep aid. If you are someone who can have a drink or two and sleep soundly, I say more power to you. I will agree that a glass or two of wine at bedtime probably helped me go to sleep more easily some nights. My problem was that I would then awaken during the night even more frequently than normal. Additionally, at this stage in my life, I would always have a hangover the next day even with just one glass of wine. Everything I have read regarding the use of alcohol states that while the use of alcohol may stimulate the onset of sleep, the quality of sleep diminishes. The usual result is frequent awakenings leaving you feeling less than refreshed the next day. On the other hand, my dentist reports that he drinks a glass of wine every night of his life to go to sleep, sleeps soundly, and awakes the next morning feeling refreshed.

I have also had people tell me stories about the use of alcohol that are similar to experiences others have with sleeping pills. A glass of wine initially may have been all that it took to help them sleep. Then they found that it took a second glass and ultimately more to achieve the same results. A point is reached when, even with increased levels of alcohol, a tolerance is developed, and alcohol no longer is of any use in getting to sleep. Coupled with a decreased quality of sleep to begin with, the use of alcohol becomes totally negative. Obviously, drinking too much alcohol is a whole new problem. I have also had people tell me that, like my night eating disorder, they have a craving for alcohol that seems to be triggered as they become more sleepy late in the evening. Furthermore, some say they will wake up and have a drink of alcohol just as I would eat a snack after sleeping for some period.

The following post illustrates what some will do to achieve a good night's sleep. I am certainly not recommending this.

Posted by * on January 21, 1998 at 15:42:09:

In Reply to: Chronic Insomnia going on 4 months! (HELP) posted by * on January 19, 1998 at 11:20:27:

I know exactly what you're going thru - support and empathy. I've recently taken to using a homeopathic medecine based on Valerian - try your local big-time health-food shop. I exceed the dosage and take it with a good stiff whisky!
When I've been trying to get to sleep, I've disciplined myself to stop trying - sometimes, I've gone for 36-40 hours without sleep...but the payoff comes when I do finally make - usually 24 hours too late!
Hang in there: the hardest thing to do is avoid worrying

Herbs and Other Supplements

As far as I know, there is no magic potion that can miraculously cure your sleep problems without some sort of side effect, tolerance, dependence, or withdrawal problems. This does not apply just to prescription medication. I hear and read more and more that people feel they can take herbs without worry. After all, herbs are natural. Everything that I read and hear about herbs gives me the impression that they act upon the human body in much the same way that prescription medicine does, which means that an educated decision should be made by weighing the benefits against the disadvantages of usage. Like prescription medicine, some people can tolerate herbs better than others. And just like prescription medicine, herbs should not be used to treat insomnia problems should never be treated with herbs other than on a short-term basis. I am aware of no studies that show that the taking of herbs on a long-term basis is safe.

There are herbs for every ailment or malady known to man. Some people swear by herbs for a good night's sleep. Some of the same people will relate later that, while there was marked im-provement when the herb was first taken, the insomnia ultimately returned. Sometimes it became worse than the original insomnia. There is no doubt that there can be serious medical consequences from the misuse of herbs. Some of those who use herbs to en-hance sleep relate worsening side effects as the dosage of the herb had to be increased. To top it off, there is very little regulation of the industry at the current time. With the lack of quality control, it is impossible to be assured of the dosage and purity of the product being used.

Subject: Re:Insomnia{Sleepless in Boston}
From: * (Rac)
Date: 1997/03/19
Message-ID: *

hi All:
Yesterday, I purchased a bottle of Valerian Root capsules. I took 4 last night{475mg each}, per suggestion of clerk, no sleep! Does this Root take time to get into one's system, or does it simply not work for me? Is the "herb" route for some, and not for others? Melatonin does nothing for me either.
Any advice on overcoming insomnia woukd be greatly appreciated, especially since it's been going on for years! I've done the sleep labs, clinics, Drs. ect!

Thanks in advance!!
Ron {Rac}

Subject: Re: St. John's Wort , Mood Enhancer (Question)
From: *
Date: Mon, May 4, 1998 23:54 EDT
Message-id: *

Yes i did try st johns..i herd so many wonderful things about
it. But like all drugs not all is for everyone. It made me very
moody and on edge all the time I quit taking it sorry i cant
help ya.
*

Subject: Re: valerian
From: *
Date: 1996/07/25
Message-ID: *

I am also a chronic, hard-core insomniac, and it did not help
me. It does smell AWFUL, and it really upset my stomach.

The following is a list of herbs that reportedly aid the sleep
process along with the reason they are supposed to help:

- Black Cohosh: For sleeplessness due to PMS.
- Chamomile: A sedative helpful for anxiety and sleeplessness.
  Relaxes digestive and nervous systems.   Relieves muscle
  cramps.
- Ginseng: Eases stress, tension, and depression.
- Passion Flower: Lowers hyperactivity and assists sleep.
- Kava Kava: For headaches and nervous tension. For
  depression-related sleeplessness.
- Hops: A flowering vine useful for soothing nervousness and
  easing headaches and anxiety

- St. John's Wort: For depression. For depression-related sleeplessness.
- Valerian Root: Settling effect on the nervous system. Aids indigestion as well as muscle cramping.

I consulted with someone in the industry who would like to remain anonymous. He related to me that the main problem in the industry is that there is no way to be sure of the exact dosage to be ingested by the consumer because the material has not gone through the purification process that pharmaceuticals do. The pharmaceutical industry is standardized. With herbs not being regulated, matters are totally different, permitting "unscrupulous people in the industry" to add "filler" to the product. He went on to tell me that herbs have chemical properties just like drugs. He said too many people do not do their homework and try an herb just because they hear someone on television talking about it. He went on to tell me that the industry, which is still in its infancy stage, is rapidly adapting to standardization of dosage like the pharmaceutical industry.

Another substance that is often touted as being a cure for insomnia is GHB. Recently GHB (Gamma Hydroxy Butyrate) has popped up on the drug scene as the new recreational drug replacing "ecstasy". In its natural form, GHB is found in every cell of the body and considered to be a nutrient. GHB is being promoted as a a medicine, sleeping aid, growth hormone stimulant, and as an aphrodisiac among other claims. It is also one of the date-rape drugs. Legally, it cannot be sold in this country unless it is under the guise of research. In addition to the legal situation, much more needs to be learned about this substance before it is tried as a sleep aid.

Impact of Medications on Sleep Stages

There are four stages of sleep and a REM stage that your body can go through each night. These stages can be repeated in cycles up to four to six times during the night. Stage one is the transition period sleep characterized by a decrease in body temperature, a slowdown in brain waves and heart rate, the relaxation of muscles, and a change in breathing to a more shallow state. This stage of light sleep can last from very few seconds to ten minutes. When awakened from stage one sleep, most people are not even aware that they have been asleep.

Sleep in stage two is deeper with most people now realizing they have been asleep even though it is relatively easy to awaken the person. This is the stage of sleep where sleepers spend most of their time. Stage two has some restorative value for the body. After the first few cycles of the night, sleep alternates between stage two and REM for the remainder of the night. It is still relatively easy to wake someone from this stage. Middle of the night awakenings many times occur in this stage.

Stages three and four are called delta sleep because of the delta waves that can be recorded on a electroencephalogram (EEG). These are the stages where the majority of the body's repair and restoration work is done. More time is typically spent in these stages after periods of strenuous physical activity. The sleeper is very hard to awaken in these stages, and, in fact, may not remember being awakened. Poor sleepers do not spend as much time in stages three and four. And while a young child may spend significant time in stage four, an elderly person may not reach stage four and may only spend a short time in stage three.

The REM (rapid eye movement) or dream stage of sleep is thought to be critical for mental restoration and the sorting out of the day' problems. More time is spent in this stage after extended periods of study or learning. The first REM stage of the night can be as short as five minutes with each return to this stage progressively longer. The last stage of REM can be as long as thirty minutes to an hour. Accordingly, most of your REM sleep occurs later in the night. The REM stage occurs about every ninety minutes and occupies about a quarter of your sleep.

In addition to the side effects that we have discussed from the sleep aids in this section, each has a direct impact on various stages of sleep. Alcohol, sleeping pills, and tranquilizers all impair the amount of sleep you get in stages three and four when the overnight repair of your physical being takes place. Marijuana, as well as tranquilizers and sleeping pills, impairs the amount of time in REM sleep, possibly affecting learning and memory functions. I have read varying accounts of the effects of aspirin on sleep. One report stated that aspirin impaired the amount of sleep in stages three and four, while another study found that aspirin aided the sleep process without disturbing the quality of sleep in any of the stages. It is important for you to monitor your reactions to the use of all substances when deciding to continue that particular sleeping aid.

CHAPTER SEVEN

Health

Long Term Use of Sleeping Pills

Nothing I have ever read recommends the use of sleeping pills for anything other than a short term solution to a sleeping problem. Why, then, do we all know people who take sleeping pills every night of their lives? Ask any pharmacist, and you will find that many people take sleeping pills for prolonged periods of time. Why are these people being prescribed this medication for extended periods? I believe the answer is that their doctors are aware of no acceptable solution other than to dispense pills. The doctor knows that his patients have to sleep. Most personal physicians do not have the time, nor probably the knowledge or the training, for the counseling and support necessary to implement behavior modification programs for their patients with insomnia. Furthermore, they probably feel as though their patient will just go to another doctor for the pills if they do not prescribe them. So with nothing better to offer than a visit to a sleep center or a psychologist for counseling, a sleeping pill is prescribed. Then the dosage is increased as the patient's tolerance builds up. The final result is that the patient cannot sleep, even with the pills. The insomnia can end up being much worse than if the medication were withheld. Sleeping pills are not the answer to chronic insomnia.

Posted by * on November 06, 1997 at 16:26:08:

In Reply to: Feels like I'm at the end of the line!!! posted by
* on November 05, 1997 at 06:15:32:

I've found that every kind of sleeping pill ends up making me
feel worse than not sleeping, I get strong side effects and little
else. As you say pills aren't the answer but I had some
success with low doses of anxiolytics plus
breathing/relaxation. I know it's possible to feel very low
because of insomnia rather than vice versa but I'm certain it's
not lasting.

Insomnia

Posted by * on December 11, 1997 at 12:27:20:

For the past 5 years I have had a severe case of insomnia
which has led me to states of anxiety which has lead to fitful
nights of terrible sleeplessness. For the last 3 mos. I've been
sleeping well on 3 mg. Klonopin along w/150 mg.Elavil.
This combo has worked extremely well. I have tried
countless other meds.but this is the best! The trouble is now
I'm having insomnia again. It's like I've become resistant to
these meds. Is this possible?
I've been to countless Doctors and Therapists and am sick
and tired(and broke). I think this problem is chemical in
nature. Do you agree? If so what is your advice. Thank you
very much.

There are several terms that we are all somewhat familiar with
that may be appropriate when a sleep medication is prescribed.
Once many medications are used regularly for even a short period
of time, there can be a loss of effectiveness due to adjustments
made by the user's body known as tolerance. Increasing doses of
a medication are necessary to sustain the initial effectiveness the

drug produced. While a sleeping medication may work in the short term, the dosage must be increased or a new medication must be substituted to produce the same results. Ultimately, the insomnia can return even with the continued use of the medication, plus there is the very real possibility of drug dependence. Withdrawal symptoms, including rebound insomnia, can occur when the sleeping medication is discontinued. With rebound insomnia, many times sleep can actually be worse than it was before taking sleeping pills.

Subject: Nothing induces sleep for me!!
From: Laura A. (Landra31@aol.com)
Date: Wed, Feb 18, 1998 15:40 EST
Message-id: *

Can anyone lend me some advice for my chronic and severe
sleep disorder? I am now 31 years old, and I have had
chronic and reocurring insomnia since I was approx. 8 years
old, however, it has become far worse in the last 3 years. It is
unbearable because I can't hold down a job for lack of sleep.
Also, I have become addicted to benzodiazapines;
(temazepam,AKA: Restoril) and even these pills are only
lending me a few hours of sleep.
I am beyond worried about my progressing and distressful
situation.

Sleeplessly Yours, Laura A.

Subject: Re: Insomnia
From: tnjayjay@aol.com (TnJayJay)
Date: 1997/08/08
Message-ID: *

I've been on the Klonopin for a month now and have had no
RLS symptoms whatsoever, it's been like a miracle, but for
the last week or so, I have had a terrible time getting to sleep.
The first week or so that I was on the Klonopin, it made me

very sleepy, but then that stopped. Once I do get to sleep, I
sleep the entire night, it's just the problem with getting to
sleep that I've got now. I'm only averaging about 3 hours a
night and having a hard time getting up in the morning.

Jodi

Smoking

Since I had smoked two packs of cigarettes a day for twenty
years, somehow the term "addictive personality", mentioned earlier in the text under "Benzodiazepines", might have applied in my
case. I wish I could report to you that my sleep was better after I
stopped smoking. The main change I noticed in my sleeping pattern was that I do not think I woke up as often as I had before. I
certainly no longer woke up in the middle of the night with a hack
cough or a sore throat caused by all of the cigarettes I had smoked
that day and the day before and the day before that. I was still
having problems falling asleep, but I think this was because of the
progression of my insomnia during this period. *Although I didn't
feel as though I went to sleep any better than before, it was nice
not to have to lie in bed and chastise myself for giving in to the
smoking habit once again. I had gotten that monkey off my back.
Every night I had promised myself that I would quit the next day.
I would then feel guilty when I didn't.* I also firmly believe the use
of tobacco has had a dramatic direct impact on the sleep habits I
developed over the years. And I feel certain that the previously
described "night eating disorder" was a substitution of sorts for
my former smoking habit. When I did smoke, I would light up if I
awoke for any period of time during the night. Likewise, if I
stayed awake much longer than normal, I would smoke a couple
of extra cigarettes. In spite of the fact that I do not think my discontinued use of tobacco helped my insomnia to any great degree,
the benefits of smoking cessation are well documented. You will
feel better, look better, smell better, and be proud of the major ac-
complishment of kicking the smoking habit.

Depression
(or which came first, the chicken or.....?)

I would also like to offer my opinion on depression. I don't consider myself to be "depressed", but I do have my good days and bad days just like everyone else. I will say the overall quality of my life suffers greatly when I am in a bad sleep cycle. My enjoyment of life diminishes, and I do not feel like a normal, functioning human being. I think that qualifies for at least a degree of depression. My question to you is "which comes first, the depression or the insomnia?" I truly feel that the depression, or my "bad days," is more a result of insomnia than my insomnia being a result of depression. In any event, I am sure you will feel much better mentally and physically when you have eliminated your insomnia. I find that insomnia magnifies any feelings of depression, anxiety, or stress.

I am not sure I know exactly what depression is. I know there are many degrees of depression. I have seen questionnaires that say if you answer "yes" to five of the ten questions, you have depression. All I can tell you is that if you feel you suffer from depression, you need to let your doctor know. Your doctor may be able to refer you to someone who can help you, just as he should do if a physical reason is the cause of your insomnia.

On the other hand, if your "depression" is a result of your insomnia, I think you will find, like I did, that the depressed feelings will subside once you begin sleeping normally again. There is a tendency when you have insomnia to start backing away from normal social interactions. You don't want to work where you are subject to a time clock or there are early morning meetings. You don't join clubs or volunteer any more because you are afraid you will not feel up to it for every meeting. It will be up to you, once you have eliminated your insomnia, to become active once again, or the feelings of depression may continue hampering your efforts to maintain good sleep habits.

Feels like I'm at the end of the line!!!

Posted by * on November 05, 1997 at 06:15:32:

I have had chronic insomnia now since mid April 97 .Prior to this date I was able to fall asleep and stay asleep like a pro. During exam time is the only time I had difficulty falling asleep and out of stupidity decided to take some prescription sleeping pills to help me doze off. They worked but when exams were over I could no longer sleep the way I had before. I visited my family docotr who referred me to a psychiatrist. I told him my error and he told me that I had not taken the pills long enough and in doses high enough to develop an addiction despite the fact I began to develop a tolerance to them. He believed that I was depressed even though I had no other symptoms besides difficulty falling asleep. I havce been on every drug imaginable. Elavil worked but had toomnay side effects.
Nothing elese has worked. I am now on Nosinan and I'm still up. Anybody have any success with this drug? I need help. I fear I'll never get back to normal.

Exercise

I am a strong advocate of regular exercise. I would like to work out four to five times a week. However, usually I get lazy and don't work out more than once or twice a week. Also, when my insomnia is really bad, it is hard to do much of anything, much less exercise. *My son suggested I subtitle this chapter "Trying to Sleep is Exercise Enough".* There have been periods of time that I have worked out as much as five to seven days a week. I would like to tell you that exercise has dramatically improved the quality of my sleep, but I can't. I know everything you have read says exercise will help you sleep, but my sleep was equally poor whether or not I worked out. I did find it more difficult to fall asleep if I worked out late in the day. Please remember, the intent of this section is not to discourage exercise, but only to relay my experience as it pertained to my sleeping pattern.

> *I have never taken any exercise except sleeping and resting.*
> -Mark Twain

> *Sleep is important. It helps reduce the risk of exercise*
> -Unknown

There is no question that I have derived some other very positive benefits from working out. As I told you previously, I have had some problems with an elevated blood pressure. Since I have always shied away from medications, I try to exercise and watch my diet every time my blood pressure gets into a warning zone. Almost without fail, my blood pressure will come back to normal levels after the exercise and diet. Furthermore, I always feel better about myself in general when I exercise regularly. On those days that I feel the worst, exercise will pick me up dramatically. Furthermore, I become better toned, look better (that's a relative term), and even lose weight if I watch what I eat in conjunction with the exercise. There is also a significant amount of healthy social interaction at the club where I work out which helps my overall mood.

General Health

I have read varying opinions as to the impact of poor sleep on one's overall health. I think one of the most important ideas to remember is that having a bad night or two will not have much of a negative impact on your performance the following day. So, if you are lying in bed at 2:00 in the morning, don't start worrying. You will be fine tomorrow. Start to accept the fact that, even though we (you and I) are going to help you, you will have an occasional night where you will not sleep well. You will call on your adrenaline supply a little more than normal the following day, but your fatigue after one night will not be that bad. The problem will be worse if you worry too much about the lost sleep. Worrying will make it harder to fall asleep at all. Any sleep and rest that you are able to get will help you tomorrow, so don't get so stressed that you end up getting no sleep. There is no question that, if your insomnia lasts over a period of time, your performance will ultimately start to diminish. But you can survive with a bad night here and there. JUST DON'T WORRY.

Some books and articles on insomnia that I have read indicate there are no long term medical consequences from lack of proper sleep. The most commonly held belief is that your immune system suffers, and you will be more susceptible to viral infections. In my case, when I am going through a bad sleep cycle, I have a much greater tendency to get sick. I am more prone to getting a sinus infection when I become too worn down. Although there have been many nights where I lay around worrying about whether my body or mind was going to suffer damage due to my lack of sleep, I have read nothing to substantiate these concerns. *Since my initial draft, I have found quite a bit of information relating to longer term health consequences as a result of insomnia. Some of this information can be found in "A Note To Readers" at the beginning of this book.*

Based on my experience, I do disagree somewhat as to ongoing health problems. There is a history of heart trouble in my family, and I have borderline blood pressure problems. On the days after I don't sleep well, particularly when I am going through a bad cycle, my blood pressure will run higher than normal. While my normal blood pressure might run 135/88, when I am tired it may run 148/97. Also, my resting heartbeat almost always runs higher during these bad cycles. While my resting heart rate may be 75-80 normally, it can be as high as 100 when I am extremely fatigued. I know it can be argued that this conclusion is not substantiated because I was not in a controlled clinical environment. I will simply submit the information as a personal opinion of the effects of sleep loss rather than a fact. I will offer this. It is currently 10:30 in the morning. I just measured my heart rate at 64. *Amazing*!

Subject: Re: Long term effects of Insomnia
From: *
Date: Fri, Feb 20, 1998 21:26 EST
Message-id: *

I think Stephen King said it best..."The death
certificate never states cause of death as insomnia. It
always says suicide." (taken from a quote from the
Stephen King novel, <u>Insomnia</u>)

Another health concern, as I have stated earlier, is that I tend to eat quite a bit more when I am really tired. I am now about twenty-five pounds heavier than I should be. When I am this heavy, not only does my back give me more problems, but my blood pressure tends to run higher. Again, it seems like my will-power diminishes after insufficient sleep. Also, it is hard for me to stay as busy when I am exhausted from no sleep, so I end up eating more when I have idle time.

The purpose of the preceding section was not to bore you with my personal life. I think it is beneficial if you will take the time to look back over your past and try to determine those things that led to your current situation. In any event, my insomnia became so bad at a point seven weeks ago that I was determined something had to change. I could not continue the way I was going. Life was absolutely passing me by.

Life can only be understood backwards; but it must be lived forwards-Soren Kierkegaard

Part III

THE SOLUTION

In this section you will be led step by step through the process that enabled me to end my insomnia. In order to receive all of the benefits, it is essential for you to read and understand each of the steps before you move forward. Consider this your prescription for your insomnia, and anything less than the total dosage will re-sult in less than desired results. Skipping ahead will result in missing a piece of the total puzzle that you need to end your insomnia.

CHAPTER EIGHT

The Plan

I. Look in the Mirror

Before you can treat your sleep problem, you need to understand insomnia and what has caused your problem. Insomnia, for
our purposes, is the inability to go to sleep and stay asleep during
the night, creating problems with functioning normally the next
day. You should not be worried about an occasional night or two
that leaves you feeling a little tired. Webster defines "insomnia"
as "prolonged and abnormal inability to obtain adequate sleep".
Again, if you have insomnia caused by some identifiable underlying problem such as sleep apnea or some medication that you are
taking, this solution is not for you. This is for those of you that
have gone to the doctor and ruled out those factors. Your doctor
might have given you some sleep medication as a short term solution and offered several other suggestions to help you. Your insomnia is not any better and, as a matter of fact, is getting
increasingly worse. *Why me*? Why in the world do you, of all
people, have insomnia? Is this another problem that you can lay
off on your ancestors who passed along your wonderful genetic
composition?   I am sure genetics are a big part of the problem.
But if you are going to cure your insomnia, you first should go to
the mirror and become acquainted with the person you see there.
You created the habits that are causing your insomnia, and you are

going to get rid of those habits. You are going to do this easily and without drugs. You will start feeling better almost immediately.

> *Not I—not anyone else, can travel that road for you. You must travel it for yourself.*-Walt Whitman

My Sunday School teacher says we are a sum of our habits (see, I do listen to what you are saying). Let's visit Webster again. Webster has several definitions for "habit" including "mental makeup; a settled tendency or usual manner of behavior; a behavior pattern acquired by frequent repetition or physiologic exposure that shows itself in regularity or increased facility of performance; an acquired mode of behavior that has become nearly or completely involuntary, addiction". Face it. You are exactly what my teacher says. All of those little habits that you have been developing over the years, good and bad, are what make up the person you are today. And the habits you have developed pertaining to sleep are what currently constitute the makeup of your insomnia, which is now also a habit. You presently have a way to treat your problems, and it is going to be easy to break your insomnia habit. *You started all of this, now put an end to it.* No, I am not going to suggest that you take a pill or eat some special food prior to bedtime that allows you to go right to sleep and sleep all through the night. But the solution is that easy.

> *Life is not the way it is supposed to be. It is the way it is. The way you cope with it is what makes the difference.*-Virginia Satir

II. Examine Your History

By reading this book you are already taking the first step toward ending your insomnia. The next step you should take is to examine your past and try to uncover those things that have occurred over the years that have left you with such poor sleep habits. In the previous section I went through a personal account of those things that I recall which caused my current inability to sleep. If you skipped over that section and came directly to the solution, it is important for you to go back and read it.

You should look at your past the same way I did. Self examination will give you great insight into how your habits developed and help you realize how a series of events over the years shaped your sleep. Even though I had already found my "cure" for insomnia when I examined my past, it was still very enlightening for me to go back while writing this book and look at the bad habits I had formed. This enabled me to realize that the steps I have taken to cure my insomnia were correct.

Next, sit down with a pen and paper or at your computer and take the time to write a sleep biography detailing from childhood everything that has affected your sleep habits. I think you will find it beneficial to write this out in a narrative format like I did. In the Appendix, I have attached a section called "Sleep Biography" that will provide questions to get you on the right track for writing your biography. At the very least, jot down some notes as you examine your past. *In order to treat your insomnia, I need your assistance. You will not be as likely to succeed if you will not take the time to complete this most important step.* I found the best time for me to write this biography was late at night when I would otherwise be trying to kill some time until I felt drowsy enough to fall asleep. You will find this is a somewhat boring task that will take your mind off the immediate worry of falling asleep, thus allowing you to become sleepy. (See the book is working already). You may not prefer to work on your biography late in the evening. Determine a time that works best for you and allot a certain amount of time per day to the writing until the biography is complete. In writing my biography, I learned a great deal about myself. You will realize two benefits as a result of this self examination. First, it will open your eyes (later hopefully closing your eyes for sleep) to the things you have done to wreck your normal sleep patterns. Secondly, if you write late at night, you will get sleepy and probably end up falling asleep earlier than you might have otherwise. My son used to joke that the reason I fell asleep more easily when I read "sleep disorder" books is that they were so boring. In reality I am sure what he said had a lot of truth to it. Reading, and likewise writing, about sleep keeps your mind off more stressful thoughts, such as worrying about actually going to sleep.

The very fact that you take the time to write your biography shows that you are serious about eliminating insomnia once and for all. You want to do whatever it takes to have a normal sleep pattern...as long as it is not too tough...and it's not. Feel free to write this biography concurrently with the start of your treatment.

"Wait a minute," you say. "Is this just another one of those self-help books that never seem to work?" Remember, I slept better from the first night. Since I have started my "cure", my sleep is better than it has been in many, many years. I say that insomnia, however ingrained, is nothing more than a bad habit. Even though the cause may have come from some very real stimuli, it was your reaction that helped form your bad sleeping habits. Are habits simple to break? If you truly want to cure your insomnia problem, you will find the steps you need to take are very simple and painless. Does it take a lot of willpower? Some willpower is required, but common sense and discipline are the true keys to success. Is that too much to ask of yourself in return for leading a normal sleep life again? Let's move on.

> *Do it now. You become successful the moment you start moving toward a worthwhile goal.*-Unknown

III. Sleep Diary

If you have ever smoked and tried to stop, one of the first things that is recommended is that you keep an ongoing journal of your smoking and the behavior that affects your habit. Now, you are going to do the same with your insomnia problem. However, just because I mention smoking, do not associate insomnia with tobacco addiction. When you stop smoking, many changes occur in your body that temporarily cause you to feel uncomfortable due to withdrawal from the drug addiction. **When you eliminate your insomnia, only positive things occur**. You feel great, you have much more energy, and you develop a more positive outlook on life.   Maybe your insomnia had caused your feelings of depression. In any event, using a journal is a proven method in breaking any addiction or habit. Like your sleep biography, your diary further reinforces your determination to end insomnia.   It also helps you to further analyze those factors that contribute to your insomnia. When completing your sleep diary, zero in on those things from your biography that you suspect impede your sleep. Experiment.

As I know you are anxious to start sleeping better immediately, feel free to start using the techniques in this plan concurrently with keeping your daily sleep diary and biography. You can start tonight with the treatment and begin the diary in the morning. *It is very important to take a few minutes each morning to complete your sleep diary. Do not procrastinate. You will find it very difficult to remember what happened exactly if you start falling behind. You need to record immediately the variables from the preceding day, how you slept, and what factors impacted your quality of sleep.* Others may have you keep your sleep diary a week or two before changing your habits to make sure you are ad-dressing your specific problem. I am confident that this plan will help you from the start. Even if you determine, after examining your sleep habits, you don't need my plan, the worst that will hap-pen is that you will end up taking a better look at yourself and your sleep habits.

Your sleep biography and sleep diary should help you recog-nize most of the reasons for your insomnia. While the use of alcohol or some sleeping medication at bedtime may help you go to sleep, you may discover their use probably hinders the overall quality of your sleep on the nights you take them. You may find late night snacks generally are not beneficial to a good night's sleep. What you are trying to discover is any kind of pattern that you can modify that is currently causing you to lie awake. You should be able to use common sense to change those habits which are negative. You may find that you are getting more sleep than you actually believed. If you perform your duties the next day without fatigue, you are probably getting enough sleep and should not be concerned. Do not worry if you are getting less sleep than you previously did, or be concerned that you now wake up a couple of times during the night. As long as you are well rested the next day, there is not a problem unless you needlessly worry about the change in your sleeping pattern. However, if you are having problems, you will learn to sleep "normally" once again in the following sections.

---

waking up twice at night

Posted by * on December 01, 1997 at 17:36:01:

The last several months I have fallen into a routine of waking up twice;always twice during the night . I have no trouble falling asleep. I can sometimes fall asleep in a matter of minutes. After waking up during the night I have no trouble falling back to sleep though not as quick as when I first fell asleep. I am 52 and even with waking up I do not feel fatigued in the morning.I realize sleep patterns change as you age but, hey if someone can give me any advice go for it. Thanks

---

Do not let the sleep diary be a burden. It should only take a few minutes. You do not have to go into great detail. I have continued to keep my sleep diary with my "cure" now in the seventh week. It will help keep you focused on good sleep habits and sticking to the plan. I also use the sleep diary to scold myself when I cheat. My next night's sleep is almost never as good if I cheat on the plan, and I use the diary to remind myself of that fact.

IV. Forget Your Existing Remedies

The initial problem that created your insomnia may or may not still be present. What has gotten worse over time is the actual insomnia itself. You have tried to deal with insomnia logically. Whenever you do not get a full night's sleep, you try to catch up on your lost sleep either by sleeping in the next morning, taking a nap, or going to bed earlier than usual the next night. It makes sense that, in order to relieve your fatigue, you need to replace the sleep you have lost. You probably have resorted to having a drink or taking some form of sleep medication. You may figure that exercise is the answer, and you do feel better, but the insomnia remains. What you are sure of is that whatever you are doing has not solved the problem. Now is the time to let go of those old remedies and use one that works.

> *I hate it when my foot falls asleep during the day because that means it's going to be up all night.*-Steven Wright

V. The Answer, Part 1 (...early to rise, makes a man...)

Now listen very, very carefully. The next three steps explain what is required to break your current pattern of insomnia. This is all you need to do. It is all so very simple. If you think about what I am going to tell you and examine your past history and current bad habits, it will all make perfect sense. It works! Trust me! I have been through hell and back, and I confidently, without reservation, tell you "It works!" For best results, however, you should write your sleep biography and keep a current sleep diary. The diary and biography do not have to be written first but can be done at the same time as the following.

First, determine what time you should wake up every morning. *It works.* If you report to a regular job outside your home every day, determining the time you should get up should be very simple. Then, get up at the same time every day, seven days a week. This will be known as your "Designated Wake-Up Time". Like to stay out late and sleep in on the weekends? If you don't have a problem with insomnia, you can do that. However, I figure if you are reading this book, you do have a sleeping problem. So listen to the answer. *It is not that hard.* How many nights have you lain awake praying for an answer? Well, here it is. *Get out of bed at the same time seven days a week and enjoy life!* In my case, I have worked out of my house for the last eight years. In the past if I didn't go to sleep until five in the morning, I allowed myself to sleep in a little (sometimes a lot) later the next morning so I would be able to function somewhat better for the remainder of the day. *Wrong!* I was still wasted during the day, and sleeping late only made sleeping the next night that much harder. *No matter how little sleep you get the night before, get out of bed at the same time the next day. Even if you get no sleep at all, get out of bed at the same time.* Most of you probably have done better than I have getting up at the same time each morning, with the possible exception of weekends. You might find that you also have what is referred to as Sunday-night insomnia. This is a condition which is characterized by sleep problems on Sunday nights after staying up later on Friday and Saturday nights and sleeping later on the weekend mornings. Once again, our good friend known as our circadian rhythms is reported to be the culprit. Any changes to our normal sleeping pattern further complicate keeping our body clock set correctly. The problem is further compounded if you take naps on the weekend. Then you can't understand why you can't get to sleep on Sunday night. Just start getting up on Saturday and Sunday mornings at the same time you do during the week and cut out the naps. *You are trying to cure your insomnia. You caused it by getting into bad habits. You will benefit if you change those habits.* Remember my father-in-law, from the "Introduction" of this book, who got up at the same time every day. Follow the example of people like him. They have developed good sleep habits.

VI. The Answer, Part 2 (less time in bed?)

Now what I am going to tell you is the key to everything. Determine how much sleep you really need to be functional the next day. What is the <u>minimum</u> amount of sleep that you need to wake up and perform life's duties without your performance being compromised? This does <u>not</u> mean the minimum number of hours that you would <u>like</u> to sleep. Later in your recovery, you will be able to spend more time in bed. But in the early days, I want you to determine the minimum number of hours that will allow you to still function properly the next day. This will leave you feeling somewhat sleepy, but nothing like the insomnia-induced fatigue that you have been experiencing. For the majority of you this will be between five and six hours. Should you make a mistake in this initial calculation, I would rather you underestimate the amount of time you need in bed. Do not think that eight hours of sleep (the amount most often associated with a "normal" night's sleep) is your norm nor the benchmark from which you should start. Do not think that, because you used to need seven hours of sleep to feel fully rested the next day, the same is true today. Besides, we are not trying to determine what will leave you fully rested at this point. Your sleep requirements can change, so don't make any assumptions based on past requirements that will cause you to worry about the amount of sleep you now need each night. Seriously consider the minimum amount of sleep that you need to get through the day. This is your "Designated Amount of Time in Bed". Later, when you have achieved some success in getting quality sleep using the times you have established, you should be able to extend your amount of time in bed. But for now, be conservative. Remember, your number one goal is not the number of hours that you spend in bed but the quality of your sleep once you get there.

The number of hours of sleep that each individual needs can be dramatically different. When I was telling my dentist that I had cured my insomnia, his assistant overheard us talking and told us that she went to sleep at 8:00 p.m. every night and slept until 7:00 a.m. This means she gets eleven hours of sleep every night ...

wow! I do not think you will find yourself needing or wanting that amount of sleep. On the other hand, there are documented cases of those that can get by with three to five hours of sleep a night. As you continue to study your sleep pattern, you may discover the only problem you have is worrying because you think there is a prescribed amount of sleep necessary each night, or that there was something wrong because you awakened several times during the night. If you find that you have good energy the next day, you probably do not have a problem. Be thankful that your sleep is as good as it is.

VII. The Answer, Part 3 (late to bed, early to rise, makes a man...)

This next part is even more important. If you set 6:30 a.m. as your Designated Wake-Up Time, and you establish six hours as your Designated Amount of Time in Bed, do not go to bed until 12:30. Let me repeat. If you establish six hours as your Designated Amount of Time in Bed, do not spend more than six hours in bed, even if you do not go to sleep when you finally go to bed. The time you go to bed, or 12:30 in this case, is your "Designated Bedtime". *I feel this is absolutely the most important thing you can do to treat your insomnia.* You will find that spending only the amount of time in bed that your body requires for sleep will assist you both in falling asleep and staying asleep. "Impossible," you say. "There is no way I can stay awake until 12:30". "Crazy", you say. "I am not getting enough sleep right now. Why would I spend less time in bed?"

Let's go to another golf analogy. Do you remember when you developed that bad slice? Everything you hit went to the right. In an effort to make a correction, you addressed the ball aiming to the left. When you went to the golf pro, he told you the answer was actually to hit the ball on an inside out path (toward the right), just the opposite of what you did in an attempt to correct the problem yourself. Aren't you doing the same thing to treat your sleep problems? It makes sense to you that, if you are not getting enough sleep, you need to spend more time in bed. So you either go to bed before you need to or you sleep late to catch up for all the sleep you have lost. And sleeping late in the morning sure feels great sometimes, doesn't it? *Well, just don't do it any more! It is the worst thing that you can do for your insomnia.*

This is where it starts to get interesting. Most of us serious insomniacs worry about the whole sleep process, particularly when we are in a bad sleep cycle. After endless nights of tossing and turning and being unable to get a good restful night's sleep, we know that the process will more than likely be repeated tonight. As bedtime nears, instead of winding down, we become more anxious. And the more anxious we become, the harder it is to fall asleep. Insomnia becomes self-perpetuating. We can't sleep, we worry about it. We worry, we can't sleep.

Here is the most important consequence that occurs when you follow the plan. You will find yourself getting more sleepy in the evenings, especially since you are starting out only getting the minimum hours of sleep necessary to make it through the day. By forcing yourself to stay awake until your designated time, you won't worry about going to sleep. Instead, it takes most of your energy just to stay awake. I know this doesn't sound right. Please let me explain. Before my "cure", I planned to go to bed anywhere from 11:00-12:30 depending on when I actually began to feel sleepy. I would lie on the couch in front of the television waiting until I would become sleepy enough to try to go to bed. Usually the closer to bedtime it got, the more awake I would become. I would finally reach a point where, even if I weren't very sleepy, I would go to bed anyway because it was "time to go to bed". Most of the time I would stay in bed for about ten to fifteen minutes and then go back to the couch. Now, because of a combination of getting up earlier every day and not letting myself go to bed until my designated time, I end up fighting to stay awake. *The pressure has been taken off to go to sleep.* I know by now you realize that a big part of your problem has been that you are so concerned about going to sleep every night that you get too anxious and try too hard. *You just have to get to sleep.* You end up tossing and turning, or you leave the bedroom and read or watch TV. You may fall asleep only to awaken, starting the game all over again. You will never get to sleep by trying harder. Sleep comes to you naturally after you develop good habits. It just doesn't work when you go to bed sooner than you should, fighting to go to sleep.

Re: waking all night

Posted by * on February 02, 1998 at 11:10:53:

In Reply to: waking all night posted by * on February 02, 1998 at 06:26:38:

Maybe it's anxiety over sleeping. I know I do the same thing. I'm so worried that I'm not going to get a good night's rest that I worry about it which makes it hard for me to get the sleep I need. I take anti-anxiety pills to help but it's really a trap because you end up getting tolerant to the medication and then it does no good unless you up the dose. It's a complete vicous cycle. the more you worry about your sleep the more you wake up in the night. Maybe try deep breathing or something that is relaxing. Good luck!

Once you start this treatment, you will get out of bed at your Designated Wake-Up Time. If it is the same time you usually get up, it will be no big deal. But for those of you who have been sleeping late, it goes against your current thinking. "I didn't sleep well last night. It makes no sense to get up now. I will be better off if I sleep another hour." *Get out of bed at your designated time! Do not break this rule. You are no longer going to be an insomniac.* Then at night you will stay up until your Designated Bedtime. If you calculated the minimum amount of sleep that you need correctly, you will find yourself fighting to stay awake. *Do not go to bed until your designated time. And if you are still not sleepy at your designated time, stay out of bed until you are.* I have read studies that say insomniacs fell asleep quicker when they were told to stay awake as long as they could. Instead of worrying about going to sleep, they concentrated on staying awake, removing the anxiety of going to sleep, and actually fell asleep earlier than normal. Again remember, the pressure to fall asleep has been removed. *Sleep will now gently embrace your body and mind rather than eluding you.*

So, what do you do to stay awake when you are feeling extremely sleepy prior to your bedtime? If you are within an hour of your bedtime during your pre-sleep routine (see below), just fight off sleep the best you can, even if you doze a little. If it is more than an hour before your Designated Bedtime, get up and walk around. Stick your head outside for some fresh air. Go for a short walk. Get yourself a drink of cold water. Do some household chores. Work on the computer. Spend extra time with your spouse and children. If you are able to snack lightly without disturbing your upcoming sleep, do so. For some, snacking works. But for those who have eating problems, snacking starts a whole new set of problems (see more on night eating in a following chapter). You are now in the process of being cured and realize you don't have to spend as much time trying to sleep, so use the time wisely. *Please pay close attention to this. If you end up spending the entire evening on the couch in an inactive state, the result will be the same as if you had napped during the day. Even if you are very tired and it is hard to stay alert, keep active. Once your sleep pattern has become more normal, you will have more energy. Get a member of your family or a friend to support you. This is especially critical in the early weeks of the plan. If you allow yourself to lie around in the evening or during the day, it will be hard for you to cure your insomnia.*

If you have any questions at all relating to your Designated Bedtime, Designated Amount of Time in Bed, or Designated Wake-Up Time, go back and read the preceding sections again. If you still have questions, please feel free to e-mail me at weed@insomniacure.com. Learn and utilize this information. These steps are essential in helping you overcome your anxiety about going to sleep, as well as improving your overall quality of sleep.

Don't treat these steps lightly. *Remember, this is the new you. You refuse to let the same bad habits ruin the quality of your life any longer.*

VIII. Pre-Sleep Routine

Very important. Develop a good regular routine prior to lying in bed that is at least an hour in length. I try to lie down on the couch in the den and either read, watch TV, or both. As we have discussed earlier, there is a strong relationship between light and your body clock, so keep lighting to a minimum at this time. I refuse to let any stressful thoughts enter my mind as I relax my body and mind in preparation for sleep. I will avoid reading or watching anything stimulating. *Reading appears to work better on those nights that I am a little more keyed up than normal or just can't seem to get very sleepy. Reading sort of puts me in another world and helps to free my mind from any distracting thoughts. For a change, I occasionally have good luck watching family videos during this time, particularly those of my boys' basketball games that I have seen before.* This is the time that you have to completely shut out all thoughts of your daily activities–past, present, and future. Many nights now I battle to stay awake during this time. Even more importantly, I now find myself ready for sleep most nights when I finally lie down in bed. I have found I do not do as well if I work late in my office and go directly to bed, even if I felt as though I would go immediately to sleep. You will find that your body needs some time to just relax and let all of the day's trauma and stress ooze out. *I would recommend that you avoid conversation during this time. You certainly don't want to get in a discussion of your financial situation or in an argument about the kids during this winding down period. However, don't shut your family off from hugging and kissing you goodnight or otherwise engaging in healthy, loving conversations.* This is especially true if you have a history of lying in bed with thoughts racing through your head keeping you awake. I still cannot fall asleep easily if I have not gone through my routine, even if I go to bed and get up at my designated times. The same thing occurs if my wife and I stay out late socially. The pre-sleep routine needs to be followed no matter how tired I may be when we return to the house.

Find a routine that works best for you and stick to it every night. Monotonous activities such as knitting are excellent. A doctor friend of mine bought a big, comfortable, rocker-recliner and lies back in it prior to bed to get ready for sleep. I had someone else recommend a rocking chair. My wife lies for about thirty minutes in a hot bath as her pre-sleep routine. She has done this for years, and, of course, has never had a problem sleeping, even with me hopping up and down in bed beside her all night. As I told you earlier, my wife convinced me of the therapeutic value of a hot bath when my legs are restless. In addition, a hot bath has the amazing ability to relax my body and mind when nothing else is working. I do not take a hot bath every night, only on those occasions when I have a hard time relaxing or foresee a problem falling asleep. I have even had success with popping out of bed when my legs are acting up for a quick hot shower directed at the back of my legs. After resorting to a hot shower, many times I can hop right back into bed and fall asleep quickly. If you have not experimented with the wonders of a late evening bath, I highly recommend that you do so. This could be just what the doctor ordered to help wash all of the days worries and anxieties down the drain, allowing you to achieve the restful sleep you desire.

Subject: Re: Can anyone help me?
From: *
Date: Sat, Feb 7, 1998 04:13 EST
Message-id: *

I had insomnia, and I cured it by listening to talk radio in bed.

*

Posted by * on November 23, 1997 at 12:58:01
In Reply to: falling into sleep problems posted by
* on November 19,1997 at 03:12:56:

one thing that I found works: playing relaxing saxaphone
music and conscentrating on it and only it until I nod off.

Posted by xxx on December 30, 1997 at 15:17:37:

In Reply to: Awake until 4am posted by * on
December 13, 1997 at 23:48:34:

* I would try taking a real hot bath about 1.5 hrs befor say
12:00 midnight for 15 to 20 minutes. Also try having
something to eat after your bath a empty stomach is no good.
when you find yourself nodding go to bed lay on your back
its also the best posistion to sleep.

The following is a little more offbeat.

Posted by * on January 31, 1998 at 15:14:30:

In Reply to: someone help me please! posted by * on January
31, 1998 at 12:31:47:

Try some incense before you sleep. It relaxed me even
though the smoke is something annoying...

I approach the pre-sleep routine like most people would their
actual bedtime. That is, I am already wearing the clothes I am going to sleep in. I have already visited the bathroom. I have turned

out all the lights and locked the doors. When I get up from the couch, the only thing I have to do is climb into the bed.

IX. Once in Bed

Relaxation Techniques

Most of the books on insomnia offer several techniques to help you to relax at bedtime. These techniques are supposed to help prepare your mind and body for a restful night's sleep by freeing your mind from distractions. Even though I had tried one or more of these techniques over the years, I basically felt they were a waste of time. Maybe they would work for the gullible or weak-willed (the same people that can be hypnotized), but my mind and body were too smart to be tricked by such simple methods (*please don't take offense to this...I am just trying to point out that I was not very open-minded*). I was way beyond getting help from deep breathing or muscle relaxation. I was concerned, however, that even with my new treatment, I might have trouble falling asleep once I lay in bed. If you recall, I had conditioned insomnia. I knew that even if the other steps worked, there was a very real possibility that I would continue my pattern of becoming aroused by the act of actually lying in bed. This was one of the last pieces of the puzzle in a cure for my insomnia, so I was determined not to be so hardheaded as to ignore professional advice. Many books recommend yoga or meditation. Others, deep breathing exercises. Others, muscle isolation. Others recommend you imagine a serene favorite place such as a lake or the mountains. And still others recommend that you imagine floating among the clouds. There are many choices that are available. You need to find one that works for you. Ask your local bookstore what books and tapes have received good feedback. Your local college or university may offer a continuing education class on yoga or some other method of relaxation. Your personal physician may have a suggestion. You will find these techniques are particularly effective on those nights when your muscles are tense and your breathing is shallow.

   This is what has worked well for me. As I lie in bed, I breathe in deeply filling my abdomen with air to a count of four or five, then breathe out slowly to the same count. As I am expelling the air, I try to relax any tense muscles. I accomplish this by concentrating on the area around my mouth, jaw, teeth, and tongue. *I want you to shut your eyes, take a deep breath, and, as you exhale, concentrate on relaxing that area now. Do this several times until you are able to isolate and relax the area.* The next area I concentrate on is around my eyes. With my eyes shut, I almost feel as though my eyeballs are trying to push out toward my closed eyelid. *Shut your eyes, take a deep breath, and relax this area as you exhale. Practice until you can feel the tension disappear.* I alternate between relaxing the areas around my mouth and around my eyes as I exhale. I repeat the process four or five times trying to relax even more with each subsequent breath. *Do the same thing when you are in bed.* Surprisingly, I find that every muscle in my body relaxes when I concentrate on the various muscles in my face, greatly enhancing the ability to fall asleep. Additionally, the sound of my deep breathing further helps me to relax by diverting my attention from other distractions.

Posted by * on November 08, 1997 at 07:15:02:
In Reply to: Feels like I'm at the end of the line!!! posted by * on November 05, 1997 at 06:15:32:

I used to have insomnia when I was younger. I started practicing breathing while laying in bed and learned to fall asleep pretty much at will and actually slept better. Now when getting to sleep becomes a problem I just concentrate on my breathing and in a couple of minutes I am sleeping. If you are interested; try making the sound you make just as you wake up in the morning. It comes from the back of your throat. I make it by sort of pushing the base of my tongue up on the inhalation and then opening the mouth slightly and making a soft "hah" sound on the exhalation. Works really well for me. I also use it in stressful situations during the day. Good luck!

Subject: Re: insomnia
From: *
Date: 1997/10/25

I have found that I sometimes have "sleepless nights," and have found relaxation tapes with some fairly comfortable headphones or "ear buds" played on my walkman to be a good solution. It doesn't bother anyone else in the house, and usually knocks me out pretty fast (I have yet to hear the end of my favorite tape in an awake state).

Although I have not tried them yet, some of the meditation techniques I have read about seem to have a lot of merit. The techniques basically involve picking a word or phrase on which you will concentrate. You are to pick some word or phrase that should not provoke any mental response from you. With your eyes closed you repeat the word silently to yourself without moving your lips. You give full attention to the actual word, not the meaning of the word. If any other thought starts to invade this process, concentrate harder on your chosen word. *If you refer to the paragraph above, it seems to me that the sound of my breathing accomplishes somewhat the same result.* Other methods include focusing on an object rather than a word. It is recommended that you practice meditation a couple of times a day for five minutes each session building until you are able to meditate for twenty minutes.

In the early weeks of my "cure", I would have nights when I did not think I needed to use these techniques. I found sleep usually did not come quite as easily on those nights. As a result, I now incorporate deep breathing and muscle relaxation as part of my nightly sleep ritual. *Don't make the same mistake that I did for so long. Muscle relaxation and deep breathing can be a major factor in completely solving your insomnia problem.*

You may find that you need to isolate other muscle groups in addition to your facial muscles in order for your body to become completely relaxed. If my method of relaxation does not work for you, try other techniques until you find one that works best for you. There are many tapes and books available on relaxation.

During the hundreds and thousands of hours that I used to lie awake in bed, unable to fall asleep, I would look for something that would provide some kind of miraculous gateway to slumber. Maybe there was a button I could push and go right to sleep. Maybe focusing all of my thoughts toward an area of my body could somehow put me out like a light. I knew it was wishful thinking, but at 4:00 in the morning, I was searching for miracles. I would have never believed anyone had he or she told me that deep breathing and relaxation of my facial muscles would accomplish what I had hoped for all those nights. Practice deep breathing and other relaxation methods until you are proficient in their use. You will also discover these techniques can be used to help you relieve stress and anxiety during the daytime. The more you practice these techniques, the more proficient you will become in reaching the desired state of relaxation.

Those with anxiety and stress related problems should find some benefit in the techniques above. If your sleep and health are being adversely affected by your lifestyle, it may be time to consider a change. Is the continuation of your current lifestyle more important than your health and well-being to you and your family? Maybe a complete change is not necessary; maybe just cutting back on your hours or learning relaxation methods will provide improvement. Quanta Dynamics, located in Louisville, Kentucky, offers the "Gift of Sleep", a program on CD for reducing stress and improving sleep. Quanta Dynamics can be reached at their e-mail address, quanta@quantadynamics.com, or by phone at 502-896-1314. Quanta's Web site is quantadynamics.com/ Quanta also has seminars available on stress reduction and sleep.

Diet and exercise are known to have a major impact on how your body handles stress and anxiety. Later, we will talk about a book, <u>Secrets of Serotonin</u>, that deals extensively with mood, depression, anxiety, and obsessive-compulsive behavior. Additionally, cognitive techniques and self-talk emphasizing more positive and calm ways for dealing with problems are suggested. A visit to a mental health professional should be arranged if you cannot deal with the problems by yourself. These professionals can train you in behavior modification techniques.

Other Aids

Many people find that the constant drone of a fan is necessary for them to find a good night's sleep. This kind of sound, called white noise, disguises other noises that otherwise might keep you awake. For some this white noise provides a calming, almost hypnotic effect. Others find the sound of a fan or other white noise disturbing and cannot be around it. Fortunately for those who share a bed, there are pillow speakers now available that allow only the person lying on the pillow to hear the sounds.

Subject: reply if the"WHITE NOISE" machine helped you.
From: *
Date: Sat, Feb 21, 1998 21:58 EST
Message-id: *

does anybody have a "WHITE NOISE" machine. If so let me know if it helped you or not   i find it hard to get to sleep at night with all the noise around me and was thinking of getting a "WHITE NOISE" machine. please email me back at *   *

Subject: Re: reply if the"WHITE NOISE" machine helped you.
From: *
Date: Sun, Feb 22, 1998 08:16 EST
Message-id: *

In the summer I find the air conditioner generates the right amount of white noise. In the winter I use an air filter for the same reason. Both work really well at blocking out street noises (and also help my allergies!).

Subject: Re: reply if the"WHITE NOISE" machine helped you.
From: art777 *
Date: Wed, Feb 25, 1998 11:05 EST

Can't sleep without it. Purchase at Sharper Image. Works great when travelling but maids make as much noise as possible to try to wake you. The maids job at most hotels and motels is to disturb as many guests as they can.

Subject: NOISE IS THE CURE!!!
From: Mrs. Ceya Minder (Robert E.)
            Dothan, Alabama
Date: 1996/07/31

My husband has horrible sleep problems...as soon as he gets in bed, he can't go to sleep or he doesn't sleep long before he wakes up and can't go back to sleep. He is from bed to couch in the den all night long.

Last year —at a garage sale—I bought a little tiny air filtering machine—just for the noise it makes. I put it beside   the bed and things are some better...but not cured.

Last weekend we were visiting my son and daughter- in-law and they had a small bubbling fountain beside our bed and would you believe....my husband slept like a baby all weekend!!! It was wonderful for him and for me.

As of yesterday, we have a small fountain beside our bed too. A simple $40.00 cure.

           Ceya

Subject: Re: NOISE IS THE CURE!!!
From: kboer@nervm.nerdc.ufl.edu (Kees Boer)
Date: 1996/08/08
Message-ID: *

I live in an apartment with a lot of university students. It can
get rowdy sometimes. I use a fan with a shirt over it. The
shirt causes it to emplify the fan noise. It works great for
cutting out unwanted sounds.

Kees

The mattress you sleep on also can be important in determining the quality of sleep that you get. I have read and heard the virtues of a firm mattress. I had always thought that a firm mattress was the choice of orthopedic specialists, although now I read that there is research supporting the use of a softer mattress. There are air and foam mattresses being offered by companies that allow your body to softly contour to the mattress resulting in less pressure being placed on the back and spine according to their marketing. If you experience back problems or any other skeletal or muscular problems, I would suggest that you at least investigate the possible use of one of these mattresses. I have not slept on any of these mattresses yet, but I have tried them in stores. I found them to feel great on my aching back which I developed spending my days in front of the computer writing this book. I would imagine they are very conducive to a good night's sleep. Even though they each utilize different technology, the following are a few companies that I am aware of that sell the mattresses:

Select Comfort Corporation
Minneapolis, MN
800-344-6561

Tempur-Pedic
Lexington, KY
800-886-6466

Relax The Back
Los Angeles, CA
800-290-2225

On the other hand, the American Innerspring Manufacturers (AIM) is a nonprofit association that provides information on healthful sleep and sleep surfaces. According to Mr. George Gwin, the associate executive director of AIM, "Through their support of numerous scientific studies and national surveys, AIM has educated a generation of American Consumers on how to get a good night's rest, as well as what to know and look for when it comes to choosing bedding. AIM funds independent studies and research on everything from sleeping patterns to spinal discomfort to purchasing patterns. We are proud to note, that all our research supports the fact that Innerspring bedding provides the best rest. Period!"

The selection of a mattress is a matter of preference. There are a great number of excellent mattresses made by a number of major manufacturers that vary according to quality and technology. You should choose the mattress that is best for you.

You can also buy magnetic mattresses that tout the relief of insomnia as one of the virtues of sleeping on a magnetic mattress. The ones I have seen are sold through multilevel marketing programs. I know very little about the mattresses other than that an acquaintance became a distributor and told me how well he is now sleeping. To say that there is a certain degree of skepticism about the validity of the claims would be an understatement of considerable degree.

Sleep Technology, located in Boulder, Colorado, just introduced (Spring, 1998) a product called the EnviroBed that is designed to eliminate light, noise and pollutants from the bedroom. The canopy-style bed is a self-contained unit covered with a ceiling, surrounded by draperies, and has its own air conditioning system for temperature control. The fan for the air is adjustable which also provides a degree of white noise and directs the air through a filter to reduce pollen and pollutants. While the bed may end up being the saving grace for travelers staying in hotels, it is available for home use also. The initial price is $3495 for the model with an air conditioner and $2995 for the model with a fan. If you have problems sleeping due to environmental reasons, this bed may be for you. The company can be reached at 303-530-0637.

Hold That Thought

Even after I had discovered my "cure" for insomnia, I was still worried about several things. My night eating disorder had improved but had not completely gone away, just as a consequence of my "cure". On occasion I would still have restless legs, which I had learned to cope with pretty well. I might have even still had leg myoclonus, though I am not sure. Another concern was the conditioned insomnia I had developed. The use of the deep breathing and relaxation techniques above have eliminated that problem for the most part. One big concern remained ... those nights when I would be totally exhausted, and my mind would still be going ninety miles an hour.

You have been there. There are nights when there is one obsessive thought which just won't leave you. It keeps going round and round inside your head, usually frustrating you because you know it is going to ruin your sleep. The thought may be job related. You may be upset because you made a bad decision in the stock market that cost you thousands of dollars. You may be concerned because the basketball coach for your eight-year-old son has not realized his star potential, but plays his own son the whole game. You may have just figured out how to get Mr. Jones to buy your company's new line of products, and you can't wait to call him in the morning. You know by now that it does absolutely no good to think or worry about these things in the middle of the night, but this just happens to be one of those nights you can't turn off your obsessive thoughts. Even worse is when you start compulsively thinking to yourself that you have to go to sleep. You cannot talk yourself into going to sleep. You must think about anything but going to sleep.

---

falling into sleep problems

Posted by * on November 19, 1997 at 03:12:56

I just can't get to sleep as I am too anxious, all sorts of questions twirl in my mind and I can't get to sleep. I thing too much and I worry too much. Does anyone have nice ways to empty your head before you go to bed? Heeeeelp! It's now weeeeeks of bad sleep that start to seriously spoil my days...

Subject: CHRONIC INSOMNIA
From: Lauren *
Date: Wed, Jan 7, 1998 19:42 EST

I've had chronic insomnia now for about 3 years. I've been to the sleep clinics, took every medication but I always end up relapsing. I'm alergic to a lot of meds, which doesn't help either. Tomorrow I'm being checked for hyperthyroidism. If anyone knows of any newer medications out please let me know. I know that if my mind would shut up at night I will sleep. But it just keeps going and going etc...... It's ruining my relationships with guys I really like because I'm thinking of them till 6:00 in the morning. I can't stop! The other night I took .5 of xanax and it didn't help one bit. I feel like my mind overpowers me. HEIP!!!!!!!!

So, what do you do? First you will find that your pre-sleep routine that I discussed earlier will be very beneficial. *I find that the time when I am lying on the couch for an hour or so serves as time to let my mind wind down. If there is something that was going to distract me from sleep, usually I can relax enough on the couch to just let the thought ooze out.* Be sure to have a nightly pre-sleep routine. *It really helps.* If you go directly to bed without your pre-sleep routine, you have a better chance of becoming pre-occupied with some thought.

If you still have thoughts banging around when you finally lie down for sleep, you will find deep breathing and muscle relaxation will help eliminate the worry many times. But there are occasions when you will still have obsessive thoughts that just won't go away, and, as a result, you will find yourself unable to get to sleep. I have found that, when I am preoccupied with a particular thought, I absolutely refuse to let the thought back in. I do everything I can to block the thought out of my mind before I get too agitated or excited. As soon as the thought comes back, I immediately begin my deep breathing and relaxation and concentrate on the sound of my breathing. There are experts who are of the opinion that you should get out of bed and write down whatever is cluttering your mind, thus bringing about some sort of closure to the subject. I have found it best not to take this approach, as I find myself getting even more worked up during that process. Without question, my best success has come by getting my mind off of the subject as soon as possible. *You have to work to develop this technique. Some people do this naturally, but it took me a while to get somewhat proficient with it. My wife likens this to a mother with a house full of kids all yelling her name. If she didn't block them out, she would lose her mind.* If all else fails, I will return to my pre-sleep routine. Oh yeah, some of my ideas really are wonderful in the middle of the night, but almost all of them don't look so great in the light of day. And yes, I have heard of songs being written in the middle of the night that became hits and of great ideas that were formulated, but I have decided a good night's sleep is more important to me at this juncture in my life. If you are able to get out of bed and get rid of the thought by thinking more about it or writing it down, more power to you. We are trying to find what works best for you.

I have developed another technique since my initial draft that works quite well for me on occasion. When I find myself stuck on some thought or continually thinking about lying awake, I mentally sing a song to myself. I have found that many times concentrating on the words of a song will free my mind enough to fall asleep. Again, strive to find what works best for you.

Still Nothing Works

There have been occasional nights since I began my "cure" when I still didn't get to sleep after getting into bed, even when I was sure I had been ready for sleep. I try not to lie in bed more than fifteen or twenty minutes before returning to the den, if I can't get to sleep. *I have found it is sometimes easier to be lazy and to continue lying in bed. Do not make the same mistake that I have. Lying in bed, tossing and turning, serves no beneficial purpose. You only stay awake that much longer, worsening your conditioned insomnia.* During this time I do not get overly concerned about not falling to sleep immediately. I just try to relax and resume my pre-sleep routine, watching television, looking at videos, or reading one more time to help me sleep.. I may take a hot bath or shower, even if I have already had one. I will use deep breathing and relaxation on the couch to help me further relax. *Remember, this is the new you. Your sleep is getting better, and even if you have one bad night, tomorrow will not be that bad. Just relax.* Then, when I begin to feel sleepy, I will return to bed. If I find myself still on the couch an hour later still seemingly awake, I will return to bed anyway. I have found that the second time I go down, particularly if it is now about an hour later, the deep breathing and relaxation will help me get to sleep quickly even though I didn't think I was ready for sleep. If you find yourself still unable to go back to sleep, repeat the process.

The good people sleep much better at night than the bad people. Of course, the bad people enjoy the waking hours much more.-Woody Allen

Subject: insomnia: can't get to sleep
From: thumps@mail.utexas.edu (Brian Tompkins)
Date: 1997/02/05
Message-ID: *

I have massive trouble getting to sleep almost every night. I'm really getting sick of it, and I've had it for about a year. It takes me about 2 or more hours to get to sleep, at least an hour on a good night. It makes me jealous hearing my friends talk about getting to sleep in 10-20 minutes. I can't remember what that's like! When I have trouble I've been alternating among melatonin, valerian(doesn't really work), and a couple of over-the counters like Diphen. Citrate and Doxylamine Succinate, just antihistamines I guess. They all work okay to some degree, but I really don't like taking things to help me sleep. I want to figure out how to get to sleep without 'outside' help. I guess my main problem is I need to learn when I won't be able to sleep instead of tossing and turning for 2 hours and wasting all that time. That's what really irritates me. Just curious about suggestions. I haven't been to a doctor, but I've tried a couple of common sense things, like cutting caffeine from my diet and trying to set a regular sleep and wake up time.

-Brian

Trouble Staying Asleep

"Okay," you say. "Your recommendation may be great for all of those that have trouble going to sleep, but I fall asleep quickly every night. My problem is that I wake up too many times and can't get back to sleep. What should I do?" The answer is that you do the very same thing. You may be the type insomniac that goes right to sleep every night but wakes up too many times. Or you wake up for good, hours before you desire. Or you may sleep all night, but find yourself exhausted the next day and suspect your quality of sleep was not very good. (*Right here, before I get all the sleep apneacs mad at me....trouble staying asleep and feeling exhausted after seemingly sleeping well all night can very definitely be symptoms of sleep apnea. If you suspect you have sleep apnea, by all means, take the necessary steps to get properly diagnosed.)* First of all, you need to go through the same steps. You may have to experiment with your bedtime and wake-up times even more than someone who cannot get to sleep. Just like those that have trouble going to sleep, write your sleep biography and start your sleep diary. Also, determine the minimum number of hours of sleep you require to function properly the next day. Set your times accordingly. So, why do you have to stay awake until a designated time if you don't have any problem falling asleep? I am going to have to give you an answer that I have read in numerous other books about sleep. If you only require six hours of sleep, yet stay in bed for eight hours, your quality of sleep will suffer even if you are asleep every minute. Your particular need is only six hours, so you end up spreading six hours of good sleep over eight hours. The analogy that is used is water in a container. If you put a set amount of water in a container that is flat, the water may be one inch deep. If you put the same amount of water in a larger container, the depth of the water (like the depth of your sleep) will be more shallow. You either wake up too often as a result, or even though you might feel like you slept well all night, the quality of your sleep suffered, leaving you "inexplicably" tired the next day.

Although cutting the amount of time spent in bed should improve the quality of your sleep, other causes for awakening during the night are often suspected to be the use of alcohol, caffeine, sleeping pills (or other types of artificial sleep aids), and tobacco. So, if you fall into this category, you need to discontinue the use of the substance causing your problem in addition to following the other steps in the plan. There are a couple of other sleeping disorders that can lead to numerous nighttime awakenings or a feeling of fatigue after seemingly sleeping all night, such as sleep apnea. Other physical causes might be chronic pain or stomach disorders. Additionally, restless legs and periodic movement of limbs, both discussed earlier in the text, can cause frequent arousal or interruption of normal sleep. While RLS and PLMS are often treated with medication, please remember that I do not take medications in order to sleep and have coped quite well.

Those who wake up too early the next morning are sometimes thought to have some degree of depression. *I really don't like the use of labels. Even more, I don't like the idea of labeling someone as possibly having depression just because he wakes up too early in the morning. I do want you to be aware that there is a school of thought that says depression is a possible cause for waking too early.* If after trying the cure you still have a problem waking too early, you might want to seek some professional help should you suspect depression is your problem. Another sleep disorder that can result in early awakenings is advanced sleep phase syndrome that was discussed briefly under the chapter on "Circadian Rhythms". Light therapy is sometimes used to treat this disorder.

One of the bad habits that I developed was getting out of bed every time I woke up during the night. Usually I would get something to eat or drink, which many times made it even harder to get back to sleep again. I am amazed that with very little willpower, I can many times resist the urge to get up. You will find the length of your time awake will be shorter if you do not get out of bed and engage in some activity that further arouses you. *I do realize that when nature calls, you had better answer.* There will still be those times when you try to stay in bed but eventually realize you are now becoming completely awake. In this instance you should leave the bedroom, just as you would if you had trouble initially falling asleep. Return to your pre-sleep routine without letting any troubling thoughts overtake you. *Once you are sure you are not going to fall asleep again, don't give in to the temptation to just lie in bed and hope that sleep will return. Once you are awake, it is better to leave the bedroom and repeat your pre-sleep routine.*

> *If you can't sleep, then get up and do something instead of ly-*
> *ing there and worrying. It's the worry that gets you, not the*
> *loss of sleep.*-Dale Carnegie

Although it is often difficult to pick up a book at 3:30 in the morning, I find that reading a book (not a stimulating one, of course) does the best job of taking my mind off of everything else and inviting slumber back into the night.

> *You know how it is when you're reading a book and falling*
> *asleep, you're reading, reading... and all of a sudden you no-*
> *tice your eyes are closed? I'm like that all of the time.*-Steven
> Wright

And, once again, don't ever give up on a hot, relaxing bath or shower, even in the middle of the night. *Please try not to wake the others, though.* If you are unable to go back to sleep at all, do not give in to the urge to sleep late, take an afternoon nap, or to go to bed early the next night.

CHAPTER NINE

Adjustments

If you are somewhat accurate determining the minimal amount of sleep you need to function properly the next day, you will probably find yourself struggling to stay awake until your Designated Bedtime from the first night. Your body is having to adjust to a more regular routine than before. If you find yourself still having problems falling asleep or staying asleep after a few days of adjusting to your new sleep schedule, you should reduce further the amount of time you stay in bed. Let's say that you need six hours of sleep and decide to get up at 6:30 every day. You will then have a Designated Bedtime of 12:30. If you are still having sleep problems, you need to reduce your Designated Amount of Time in Bed. Try reducing your time by thirty minutes, moving your bedtime to 1:00. If that still doesn't work, keep moving in thirty minute increments until you have found the times that work best for you.

On the other hand, if you are struggling to stay awake until your designated time, going right to sleep when you first lie down, not waking too much during the night, and still feel tired the next day, you might want to increase your time in bed by thirty minutes. In our example you would extend your Designated Amount of Time in Bed to six and one-half hours. *Please don't get lazy on me though.* Make sure any adjustment results in better quality sleep. If you extend your sleep time and the quality of your sleep diminishes, you need to reduce your time in bed once again. Play with the times until you find what is right for you. *Before you extend your Designated Amount of Time in Bed, you might want to try the following:* When I am unable to stay awake until my Designated Bedtime and give in to the urge, I will get up that much earlier the next morning. For example, if you should set your time at 12:30, but instead go to bed at 12:00, you should get up at 6:00 rather than 6:30 the next morning. You should never go down more than thirty minutes before your Designated Bedtime, nor should you exceed your Designated Amount of Time in Bed. In this example, you should never sleep beyond your Designated Wake-Up Time of 6:30 a.m. *Then, make a smart decision as to whether or not to increase your time in bed.*

As I told you earlier, I started out going to bed at 1:30 and getting up at 7:30. Once I had settled into my routine and developed some of my techniques, I realized that I could sleep a little longer and still get quality sleep. I ended up being able to stay in bed for seven hours with no problem getting to sleep and staying asleep. *If anyone had told me that I would be getting seven hours of quality sleep a night two months ago, I would have told him he was out of his mind.* I have also changed my wake up time to 7:00 a.m.. As a matter of fact, on several occasions I have gotten up even earlier. For years I have wanted to get up around 6:00 every morning. While I was still struggling to get a few good hours of sleep, I was always frustrated and embarrassed to get up at 9:00 a.m. Some people had been up and productive for hours. When I used to fish, I loved dawn with the transition between the stillness of the preceding night and the first rustlings of the birds looking for food. I look forward to the time when getting up at dawn is a part of my regular routine.

Once you have set your Designated Bedtime, stick to it as much as possible. This schedule is not meant to be set in concrete with no changes. Try to be as consistent as possible from night to night. Keep a good record in your sleep diary of the effects of any time changes you make, in addition to anything else that influences the quality of your sleep. I still keep my sleep diary daily, and I am still learning from it. How long should you stay with your designated times before you make adjustments? I would recommend waiting for at least three to four days before changing your sleep time or wake-up time.

Do not move your wake-up to a later time unless you first move your Designated Bedtime later. I would not recommend moving your wake-up time later unless there is some significant change occurring in your life, such as a job change where your hours are later, or retirement. Otherwise, keep the same wake-up time or move it earlier if it so suits you.

> *The successful man will profit from his mistakes and try again in a different way.*-Dale Carnegie

CHAPTER TEN

Support

This is the perfect time to talk about support. Like most other members of the human race, you will sometimes stumble. When you start this program, many of you will need support to get the maximum results. The most obvious place to start is with your family...your spouse, children, mother, father. Be sure to tell them what you are trying to accomplish and how you are going to go about it. Tell them you are trying to avoid snacks late at night or your evening glass of wine. Let them know how important it is for you to avoid a late night argument that could interrupt your sleep. Have them share in your successes. After all, they will benefit from your improved disposition and your increased energy level. They hate seeing you suffer when you don't sleep well.

Tell your friends you have finally found something that will end your insomnia once and for all. You will find that telling others will help provide incentive for you to succeed. Tell another insomniac. Have him go through this program at the same time. Help each other by sharing your successes and failures. Find someone you can call late at night when you are having trouble staying awake until your Designated Bedtime. Form a support group with others who want to use this plan.

Subject: Re: Can someone please help me?
From: *
Date: Fri, Feb 6, 1998 03:54 EST
Message-id: *

Hi there!

Would you believe - I had very much the same problem in
my University days - and I certainly do sympathise with you.
It is a real trap for some students - a few late nights and then
you start sleeping in, then a bit longer ..... and before you
know it, you're way out of sync with everyone who doesn't
have this sort of problem. A really rotten trap - dead simple
to fall into, but getting out?   - that's an entirely different
matter.

I missed a whole semester for 2 out of my 3 subjects in 3rd
year, because the lectures were at 9:00 in the morning.
"That's not early" most people would say, but for years and
years (16 in fact) I had great trouble waking myself before 8
or 8:30 am. I bought an alarm clock with a very loud alarm -
like a fire alarm, some of my neighbours reckoned - but all
too often the alarm ran out before it could wake me. Then
when clock-radios became available, I bought one of those,
but after the novelty wore off, I still managed to sleep
through breakfast time, radio blaring and the alarm buzzer
buzzing away.....The only solution in my situation was to
have some one come and physically waken me by shaking
me or even slapping me in the face with a cold, wet face
washer.

Lucky for me, I managed to get back on track over the
semester break. I count myself very fortunate indeed, in
having a really good friend who was prepared to nurse me
along for something like 2 weeks. He would come around
and waken me at 8:00am, and stay with me to make sure I
stayed awake, while I struggled through the day, copying out
notes for lectures I had missed, had meals, and so on, until
10:00pm when he left me alone to get some sleep. The first
few days were pretty shocking, forcing myself to stay awake
and it took a lot of dogged determination to stick to the

agreed schedule - both on his part as well as mine. A big help was the realisation that I was placing a huge burden on my friend and friendship - and so I didn't want to let his efforts go to waste. I was so grateful for his help and support - and so we stuck at it, and finally by the time the next semester started, I was back on a "normal" schedule again, Well, I still had to rely on my friend coming round to waken me in the morning, but otherwise...Doctors couldn't do much except offer a medical certificate to cover my absence on medical grounds.

Hope I've been of some help to you
Derrick

If you are religious (or even if you're not), pray for the strength to reach your goals. Have your family and friends pray for you.

I am a firm believer that my daily diary provides me with strong support. Every time I want to quit or cheat on the program, my alter ego reminds me through my sleep diary to remain strong and to discover why I am weak or what changes I need to make to continue my cure.

You can e-mail me at weed@insomniacure.com, and I will answer your questions or make arrangements for someone else trained in the program to help you. If I get enough requests, I will set up a Web page that offers support from others who are also trying to cure their insomnia.

As self-described in its Web page, "The National Sleep Foundation is a nonprofit organization that promotes public understanding of sleep and sleep disorders and supports sleep-related education, research and advocacy to improve public health and safety. Established in 1990, the Foundation relies on corporate and individual donations, and partnerships with corporations and government, to fund its many educational and research programs." Their Web address is at http://www.sleepfoundation.org/. Or you can write to:

National Sleep Foundation
729 Fifteenth Street, NW, Fourth Floor
Washington, D.C. 20005

Many of the Internet postings that I used came from a "newsgroup" called alt.support.sleep-disorder. Another site that is very helpful for insomniacs is the "Sleep Forums" located at http://www.sleepnet.com/wwwboard/wwwboard.html. This site is administered by an individual known as the Sandman. The Sandman graciously gave his permission for me to contact authors of the posts that I used from the "Forums". In addition to the "Sleep Forum" site, the home page is called "SleepNet" which was started to inform the public about sleep disorders and sleep deprivation. "SleepNet" offers a world of information on sleep disorders and strives to provide a link to all the sleep information on the Internet. The "SleepNet Forums" and the alt.support.sleep-disorder "newsgroup" both feature interaction among those with sleep disorders. Both sites can be of great assistance in overcoming your insomnia.

CHAPTER ELEVEN

Be Committed

Every Step Is Important

Okay, now you have been given the steps necessary to address your insomnia problem. The next step is up to you. You have to be committed to doing whatever is necessary to cure your insomnia. That means follow <u>each</u> of the steps presented above. *Many medications contain the instructions to continue taking all of the medication until all of the pills are gone even if you are feeling better. This is done so the illness will not return. The same is true with this program. Continue using this plan even after you start sleeping better, or the insomnia may return. If the symptoms reappear and you need a refill, all you have to do is carefully read the solution again and follow the steps.* If you are not committed to making a lifestyle change in order to treat your insomnia, then put this paper away and pull it back out when, once again, your insomnia is wrecking your life. The worst thing you can do is to approach the treatment haphazardly, picking out only one or two things that you think might help you and ignoring the other information as irrelevant to your particular circumstance. I assume the reason you are reading this book is not to read the "fascinating" life and times of John Wiedman, but to end your insomnia. Your life is being turned upside down because of the effects of too little sleep. This treatment can work for you. If you say, "I like the part about getting up the same time every day, but I have got to get my sleep on weekends", and "the sleep biography idea sounds okay, but it's not really going to help me", then put this book away. If you try to use only a part of the suggested treatment and fail, you may end up being more frustrated than before.

On the other hand, each of us is a distinct living creature that reacts differently to different treatments. I fully realize what works for me in a particular circumstance may not work for you. It is possible that your pre-sleep routine will be completely different from mine. You may only need fifteen minutes to wind down or maybe two hours. It may be that you can take a nap every day. It may turn out that you don't need to go through deep breathing and muscle relaxation when you finally lie down in bed; that these techniques actually cause you to become more aroused. So, am I backing off from what I said in the previous paragraph? No. I think each of the steps in the plan is vital to the success of the plan, but you have to make adjustments to fit your individual personality. If you can achieve a quality of sleep that is satisfactory to you by only following one or two of the steps, more power to you. But if you are still having trouble sleeping, you owe it to yourself to try the whole package. Let's say you are convinced that a daily nap doesn't affect your nightly sleep, but you are doing everything else correctly and still can't sleep well. Cut out the nap. At least stop napping for a long enough period to gauge the results, say five or six nights. You will be uncomfortable eliminating the nap for a while because it has become a habit, but the nap may indeed be the determining factor in ending your insomnia. Likewise, if you feel that you have to go to your bed for your pre-sleep routine but still can't sleep, try another room for several nights. We have got to break those old habits.

The answer you are looking for lies within these pages. Oh sure, I was just like you. I have seen all of these ideas presented in one form or another over the years. On one hand, this plan seems almost too simplistic. You feel that something more dramatic or sexy is necessary to eliminate your insomnia. A pill, perhaps ... you know there is one somewhere that you can take, and all of your sleep problems will go away, with no side effects. Or maybe a food, or an herb. How about divine intervention? Anything but behavior modification.

Subject: onset insomnia
From: Dark Force *
Date: 1997/11/26
Message-ID: *

I have a problem with getting to sleep. I will be very tierd and want to sleep but at the same time my mind seems to be racing and I just can't get to sleep. I will toss and turn for hours, finally, I give up and say up. Eventually I burn out and sleep for two days straight. Other times when I can't get to sleep I resort to sleeping pills or alcohol either which puts me to sleep but when I wake up the next moring I feel like I have not slept at all. The only difference is that at leat I was not awake all night. Has anyone had this problem??
Any advice is greatly appreciated.

> *Advice is what we ask for when we already know the answer, but wish we didn't.*-Erica Jong

But the techniques in this book do work. Why keep on being miserable day after day with the false idea that your insomnia will miraculously go away? You have to take charge. You already know that the medications you are taking don't work. None of the over-the-counter remedies are working. Herbs had worse side effects than the prescription medications, and who knows what exactly was going into your body. This is the answer. Go back to steps I and II. The answer is <u>you</u>. Don't trivialize this plan. Don't rationalize why it won't work for you. Try it. And don't give up after the first night or the second or the third or the second week. How long did it take you to develop your poor sleeping habits? If not years and years, at least months and months. Don't expect overnight miracles. And realize that as a human you are not perfect; you will make mistakes. You will give in to temptation. (I am beginning to sound like Reverend Ike.) I made some of my biggest mistakes after I had achieved a degree of success in treating my insomnia. I figured that it might be okay to go to bed early. I deserved it, and one night wouldn't possibly hurt anything. I was wrong. But it was my fault and not the fault of the plan. Stay with the program, you will see results.

Subject: Trouble sleeping
From: *
Date: 1998/01/19
Message-ID: *

Hi

It's my first time in here and am looking for any info about
trouble sleeping. I'm a healthy female who cannot fall asleep
at night. Having tried the most common things, first
sleeping pills which left me more tired in the morning than
rested, cammomile, tea, milk, etc nothing seems to work.
Some times I will be utterly exhausted and yet unable to
sleep. This has been going on for a couple of years now.
Any info will be greatly appreciated.
Thanks in advance!

Facing Adversity

Sure, I know I said I slept better from the first night. Well, I did. Does that mean I slept perfectly from the first night? No! I am constantly having to reevaluate and make changes. On the third night, I may have gotten out of bed for a couple of hours before getting back to sleep. So what! I was still way ahead of where I was the week before, and I was seeing progress. Two

weeks later I was up until 3:30. Discouraging? Sure, but I had
slept great the three nights before, so I knew I was on the right
track. After three months I had three bad nights in a row. Could
it be the program was no longer working? Of course it was still
working. Hadn't I been sleeping better than I can remember in
years? *Your body will not develop a tolerance to this plan like it
would with a pill. We are in the process of instilling new habits to
replace those old habits that do not want to go away without a
fight* My present problems compared to my previous problems
are like two six year olds fighting in the school yard compared to
World War II. (I can't remember exactly where I heard this quote,
so I cannot give proper credit.)

---

*If you get up one more time than you fall, you will make it
through.*-Chinese Proverb

When I started the program, I was totally committed to doing
the right things to "cure" my insomnia. I knew that if I did not
change my lifestyle, I would end up in the grave years before my
time. When I had a bad night, I didn't say, "This plan is not
working, I am going to have to start taking trazodone again." I
wrote in my diary, "Okay, what went wrong last night? Did I stay
in bed too long the night before? I'll make an adjustment". Or
maybe I wrote, "I slept a little later than I should have yesterday
morning. I cheated, and I had to pay for it last night. I didn't
want to get up at my designated time, but I will know better next
time". Or, "Instead of getting out of bed and reading, I thought I
could stay in bed and finally fall off to sleep. Well, I didn't, and
the next time I can't fall asleep I will get back out of bed and return to my pre-sleep routine". Or, "I know I shouldn't have eaten
that late night piece of pizza. I know from my sleep diary that I
have trouble sleeping any time I eat pizza. I will try to be stronger
next time". Or, "It was another of those nights that I just couldn't
shut down my thoughts. I have got to work on relaxation

techniques and the ability to shut things out of my mind. Maybe I will try a hot bath like the book suggested".

> *When I woke up this morning my girlfriend asked me, "Did you sleep good?" I said, "No, I made a few mistakes."*-Steven Wright

The steps in this book may seem simple when you first read them. Too simple. You and I are human beings. We have to be convinced something can work. We can tell by our drowsiness that a sleeping pill is doing something. It may not be the feedback we desired, but the results occur very quickly. When we are modifying our behavior, the results may take a little longer. It may not be very comfortable trying to stay up until the wee hours of the morning or getting up at the designated time with only a couple of hours sleep, but the results are remarkable. You may find it hard not to reach for the same bottle of pills that have failed you night after night ... you remember they did work the first night or two you tried them. You know your sleep is now worse than it was before you started taking the medication, but ...maybe tonight.

There has got to be a certain amount of trust and faith when you start this program. You have to have confidence that the program can really eliminate your insomnia. When you have seriously reviewed the events that led to your insomnia, you will realize that your habits do need modification. You have to believe in yourself, that you can be strong enough personally to do the things necessary to treat your insomnia. You have to believe in this program, that it can provide the answer you have sought for so long now. When the going gets tough, you have to be disciplined, figuring out what adjustments you have to make to end your insomnia.

> *You may have to fight a battle more than once to win it.*
> -Margaret Thatcher

Follow the Plan

Let's reexamine each step of this plan once more. When I started my cure, I had almost everything else in place except the sleep biography. I found that the more I wrote about my problem, the more committed I became to curing my insomnia. I could now see those things that I had given up as a result of my insomnia. My life was becoming a wreck. *Even my wife was more sympathetic to me after reading this for the first time ... for a while ... a very short while.* My health was deteriorating as evidenced by my blood pressure and my heart rate. The sleep biography caused me to examine the events that led to my current habits, thus helping me to overcome any second thoughts about the effectiveness of this plan. It helped me put everything else in perspective. My family was the most important thing in my life. What kind of father was I becoming? It is awfully easy to procrastinate about things in life, even those things that are ruining your life. The sleep biography helped me to recognize that every factor which contributed to my insomnia would not be changed overnight.

Keeping a daily sleep diary is essential to treating your problem. Eliminating insomnia happens <u>one day at a time</u>. Last night you didn't sleep well. Did you eat too much? Did you sleep too much the night before? Every day you must look at what occurred the night before and at what happened yesterday to affect your sleep. When you are trying to spot a pattern that impacts your sleep, you may have to go back several weeks in your diary. You may go several days in a row, and everything is perfect. You start to get a little sloppier with the new habits you are developing. Then bang! Three nights in a row of poor sleep. You now start to question whether you are getting better or not. It takes making adjustments to get your sleep pattern somewhat regular again. *I am now in the fifth month of my "cure" and have to watch myself daily so that I won't develop bad habits once again.* Do not make keeping the diary a big deal. Take a few minutes each day to track your results, examine what happened to affect your sleep last night, and fine tune "your" plan. Scold yourself if you cheated.

The steps in the plan relating to the number of hours you spend in bed, the time you go to bed, and the time you awaken all contribute to breaking your current cycle of insomnia. These steps help you overcome your anxiety about going to sleep as well as directly influencing the quality of your sleep. **If you truly are dedicated to ending your current insomnia and starting to sleep better again soon, you should follow these steps. The first thing you should do is cut back the number of hours you spend in the bed to a minimum. This step is essential to get you back on track! Everything else will help to improve your sleep habits, but you must first break out of your current pattern.**

Your pre-sleep routine, breathing and relaxation techniques, blocking out unwanted thoughts, and leaving the bedroom when you are unable to sleep are all major pieces of your insomnia puzzle. These steps help to control your racing mind as well as the conditioned insomnia you have developed. *The quality of your life has suffered. You refuse to continue the same bad habits. Your life is going to get better starting today.*

Hardest Parts of the Plan

If you are currently going through a bout of insomnia where you cannot get to sleep or cannot stay asleep, you must cut back the number of hours in bed to an absolute minimum in order to get your sleep pattern back to normal. **Let me repeat, you must go through a period of time when you cut back the amount of time in bed to an absolute minimum. You must go to bed and get up at your designated times. Every other step in the program will help you develop good sleep habits once again, but only this step will break your current trend of tossing and turning in your bed.** For some people this can be tough, but it won't take long before you start to realize the benefits of this process. *You can do this. You are ready to end the misery that is occurring night after night.*

You might have a problem popping out of bed every morning. If you are like me, you already have this problem anyway. Before my "cure", I would not require myself to get up in the morning, which in itself was a major mistake. I have had trouble getting up in the morning for as long as I remember. I will tell you this without reservation, though: Now once I have gotten out of bed and cleared the cobwebs, I feel better for the rest of the day, regardless of how many hours I have slept. My sleep the next night is almost always better if I stick to the program. But, I still have to be careful in the mornings, or I will talk myself into staying in bed for a little longer. Almost without fail, when I cheat on my program, I do not sleep as well the next night. *Please don't be foolish like I have been on occasion. The program works. Get out of bed. Sure, it feels awfully good to sleep in just for a little while, but habits like this got you in trouble in the first place.* I addressed how to make adjustments in chapter nine.

Another problem is that you will find yourself fighting to stay awake until your designated time each night. Although you had the option of lying down when you wanted to before, the plan now requires you to stay awake. I assure you this is better than your current insomnia and the subsequent problems. You will find yourself either adjusting to the new hours or sleeping well enough to experiment with spending extra time in the bed. *However, do not end up extending your time in bed where you once again do not fall asleep or stay asleep satisfactorily.*

There is a possibility that you will also feel more tired during the day for a while. You will quickly adjust to your new sleep routine. If you start to sleep well at night and still find yourself sleepy during the day, you can experiment with extending your hours in bed. Occasionally you might have a night when you do not get as much sleep. Do not give in to the urge to sleep late or to nap for a while the next day. *Sure the day will be tougher than normal, but this isn't as bad as you felt most days before you made the changes necessary to conquer insomnia. Don't give in!* If you feel the urge to nap, try going outside and walking.

The toughest part of the program probably is having the discipline to stick with it. Interestingly enough, this problem occurs both when everything is going smoothly as well as when the going gets a little shaky. You will be tempted to become complacent when you start to sleep better, forgetting how miserable you felt following night after night of insomnia. You may find yourself starting to cheat on the program. You may start to sleep later than you should or go to bed too early. If you keep up with your diary, you will be able to monitor what is happening and scold yourself when you cheat.

> *How many a man has thrown up his hands at a time when a little more effort, a little more patience, would have achieved success?*-Elbert Hubbard

On the other hand you may start to question the effectiveness of the program when you are going through a couple of bad nights. You want instant, long lasting results, and you weaken when things don't go perfectly. *Just remember, you have already seen good results when you consistently follow the plan. Recognize that your lack of discipline can nullify your progress.*

> *Instant gratification is not soon enough*-Meryl Streep

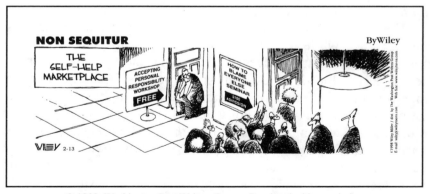

© 1998, Washington Post Writers Group. Reprinted with permission.

CHAPTER TWELVE

Retrospect

Another Look at Night Eating

By the way, right here I want to address my night eating disorder once again. This is probably the part of the book that I was most concerned about after the initial draft. The more people I let read my draft, the more I discovered that this pattern of bingeing in the evening was a somewhat common problem. I would estimate that 10 to 15 percent of the insomniacs that I have conversations with have this disorder. I would further estimate that up 20 to 30 percent have some kind of problem related to eating, interfering with a good night's sleep. Even worse, while others were looking to me for some sort of guidance, I continued to have significant problems of my own with binge-type behavior in the evenings. The cravings did not prevent me from getting to sleep as much as they caused me to feel down about my inability to control my behavior. Once again, my eating triggered my restless legs, or vice versa. Here I was telling the world how to control insomnia through changes in lifestyle, and I could not control my appetite. I received quite a bit of feedback asking for help in how to control this behavior, and I didn't really have a clue.

I would try to watch what I was eating and usually drank diet soft drinks all day to keep from eating anything else. I even tried the two-liters-of-water-a-day routine. But my real problems always started in the evenings, after dinner, when I would snack or want to snack the whole evening until bedtime. I absolutely could not stop snacking. It was like I was going through withdrawal symptoms and had to have food. Then, when I would give in and eat something, I would crave food even more. And then my restless legs problem would worsen after I had eaten. I was doing much better, though, about not eating once I had gone to bed.

I researched this area more than any other after the writing of the initial draft. I did find more and more information on the subject, though not many solutions. I did start to learn more and more about the effects of certain foods upon moods and binge eating, primarily manufactured foods that are high in fat and sugar. I also learned from differing sources that the use of artificial sweeteners was not conducive to the elimination of food cravings. I decided that maybe these authors who wrote about eating disorders knew what they were talking about. Maybe I should listen.

About ten years ago I mustered the willpower to lose a significant amount of weight. I worked out seven days a week most of the time during this period. I felt great about myself. I ate a lot of rice cakes...at the time there weren't the choices in rice cakes that there are now...and many low-cal frozen dinners. I relied heavily on artificial sweeteners and diet drinks to get me through. And although I lost quite a few pounds, every day was a bit of a struggle to keep from snacking. Once I lost the weight and started drifting away from daily exercise and started eating sweets and fats again, the weight came back. And the gain of additional weight made more exercising that much tougher. And the more I ate, the more my back hurt once again.

Recently, I finally reached the point where something had to happen to stop this vicious cycle of eating and craving. So here is what I did. I was fed up with having no control and bingeing night after night, so I decided I was going to get up but not start snacking. Was there any possibility that all of the junk I was eating was causing me to crave more? From the first morning I tried this, my cravings decreased dramatically. I intentionally tried to stay more busy than normal to keep my mind occupied and not think about food. I decided to drink ice water (no, not two liters a day) if I had any desire to snack. While I thought the ice water would help curb my hunger pains, in reality drinking it served to keep my hands and mouth busy when I became bored. I decided to drink a glass of Instant Breakfast in the morning and to have a light lunch of yogurt or tuna or fruit. Then for dinner, I ate what my family did, just smaller portions than I always had before. I drank ice water with my meals.

The turnaround from the day before and all the days before that was unbelievable. By eliminating sugars and sweets and cutting back on the fats, except those in my normal evening meal, the constant cravings to eat diminished greatly. If my family was having something that was a little too aggressive for me, like pizza, which had always triggered more eating, I might fix myself a diet frozen dinner like macaroni and cheese. I intentionally avoided most foods with artificial sweeteners, particularly diet drinks. Instead of exercising seven days a week like I did before, I started exercising three days most of the time, occasionally four days. I felt if I did not make exercise too demanding, it might be easier to sustain a regular program. I started out slowly, primarily because my hip and lower back gave me so many problems, but I did move up so that I am now jogging at least half of my aerobic routine. I don't particularly enjoy weights, so I only use them a couple of times a week. Exercise will assist your efforts to lose weight, but unless you reduce the consumption of unhealthy foods, you will never attain your goals.

I really hesitated before letting you know that I had good results with this. I already have people tell me the reason I was able to cure my insomnia was due to tremendous willpower, which is not true. Now I am telling you that I have eliminated my nightly bingeing, and some people might think it's nothing but strong willpower. Well, yesterday, after six weeks of new eating patterns, I read most of the Secrets of Serotonin by Carol Hart. The book explained exactly why I was having the success I was. I am one of those that likes to know why something is working. I was really pumped up after reading the book, knowing the reasons why the things I had done were working. *I am no miracle worker.*

You need to buy the book if you have problems with binge eating or mood swings. It's only $5.99 and, if you only read chapters eight, nine, and ten, you will be ahead of the game. *So please don't think the things I recommend to you are impossible to achieve or require superhuman willpower; they don't.*

In her book Ms. Hart points out the following:

- Why the eating of sugar can lead to the lowering of blood sugar levels and subsequent cravings for more food.
- The use of artificial sweeteners, natural honey, canned fruits, and dried fruits can stimulate appetite rather than curbing it.
- Eating personally favored foods leaves one feeling hungry faster than an alternative containing an equal number of calories.
- What foods and when to eat them to keep levels of serotonin in your body at optimum levels.
- The impact of sugar, fat, and other foods on your serotonin levels.
- The lifestyle changes that can support your new eating habits to boost serotonin levels.
- The impact of serotonin levels on your mood, insomnia, cravings, and depression.

In February of this year (1998), there was a report issued stating that scientists had isolated a "hunger hormone". They dubbed the hormone "orexin," which comes from the Greek word for hunger "orexis". The scientists reported that the brain produces the hormone when it senses a need to eat. They feel there is now the possibility of combating eating problems–both eating too much and too little. In the <u>Secrets of Serotonin</u>, Ms. Hart points out that serotonin does not act alone in the control of our mood and other behavior, but it does act as the leader in directing the output of the brain.

I like the book because of the use of alternative methods for treating depression, cravings, and insomnia without the use of prescription medicines. I am sure there are other books on the market that also explain the relationship between the foods we eat and our subsequent cravings, and I do not mean to detract from them. There are several books and diets on the market about food addictions which suggest that the eating of certain foods can trigger bingeing. I have not read any of these books, so I cannot personally offer any testimony as to their effectiveness. I have read information on the Internet from those who are following the plans and swear by them. I understand some of the findings may not be totally shared by the mainstream nutritional community. Most of the books are for the most part consistent with the Secrets of Serotonin as to what foods to avoid. As with insomnia, I like to see alternative methods of treating eating problems exhausted before medications are used. Although I am sure I am leaving out many good books, the books that I seem to hear the most about are:

> Food Addiction: The Body Knows by Kay Sheppard (she has a support discussion group on the Internet where questions about the plan are answered.)

> The Carbohydrate Addict's Diet by Drs. Richard and Rachael Heller

> Cure For All Diseases by Hulda Clark

On another note, you will hear and see a lot mentioned about the consumption of tryptophan, an amino acid, to aid the sleep process. Tryptophan is found in all animal protein including dairy products, eggs, meat, and fish. Tryptophan is also found in nuts, seeds, and some vegetables.

Foods that help you sleep

Posted by Kristina on December 16, 1997 at 20:23:00:
I have heard that there is a natural chemical in chicken that will help you sleep.. Has anyone else heard this??

Posted by Kelly zerograv@surfree.net on December 19, 1997 at 08:45:10:

In Reply to: Foods that help you sleep posted by * on December 16, 1997 at 20:23:00:

Tryptophan is naturally occurring in turkey.

Posted by * on December 19, 1997 at 13:42:17:

In Reply to: Re: Foods that help you sleep posted by * on December 18, 1997 at 06:22:57:

L-tryptophan is one of the 23 naturally occurring amino acids present in the proteins you eat that your body can break down and utilize. Poultry (especially turkey) is a protein source rich in tryptophan. The theory that has been presented is that tryptophan is a biochemical precursor to serotonin (a neurotransmitter involved in sleep and mood processes), so increase in tryptophan in the diet will lead to increase in serotonin. This has not been clinically proven. In amino acid metabolism, the body has a tendency to utilize what is available, and break down the excess amino acids into energy instead of protein building blocks. If you were tryptophan deficient, supplementation would help. A "normal" diet should provide adequate levels of tryptophan, vegetarian diets have a greater chance of deficiency unless carefully planned

---

Subject: Re: warm milk question
From: *
Date: 1997/10/30
Message-ID: *

Its Tryptophan, the same thing in Turkey that makes you want to sleep after you've stuffed yourself at Thanksgiving. It is available here in Canada as a prescription medication approved by the Canadian Health Protection Branch (Canuck FDA). Interestingly, it is illegal to sell Melatonin in Canada. Tryptophan is a Melatonin precursor.

In the <u>Secrets of Serotonin,</u> Ms. Hart points out that our bodies already have an adequate supply of tryptophan and that eating more will not result in more reaching your brain for the desired results of sleeping better or improvement of mood or cravings. However, the consumption of carbohydrates does result in more tryptophan reaching the brain where it is used to produce serotonin. The role of serotonin in sleep is still not understood. It is known that melatonin, which is made by the body from serotonin, is required for normal sleep.

The American Dietetic Association provides a wealth of information on nutrition through their Web Site located at http://www.eatright.org. They also have a comprehensive guide relating to food and nutrition called <u>The American Dietetic Association's Complete Food & Nutrition Guide</u> by Roberta Larson Duyff, SM, RD, CFCS.

I am excited about the changes that have occurred in my eating patterns. If you have an eating problem in association with your insomnia, you should explore some of the resources available to help curb your eating disorder. The best way I know to sum up the dramatic change that has occurred with me is that the fewer sugars and fats and favorite foods that I eat, the fewer problems I have with craving and bingeing later. I personally attribute my lack of cravings at this time to the elimination of artificial sweeteners as well as sugars and fats.

Sleep Clinics Revisited

The key to my "cure" is behavior modification, a word that in the past had not conjured up images of eliminating my insomnia and helping me to get a peaceful night's sleep. But it was and is the answer to my problem. From the responses I have received so far, I think most people have always been skeptical about the success of behavior modification (just like I was), particularly as to the potential of actually helping in their specific instances. They have always wanted to believe their insomnia would either go away with time, or some pill would come along that would cure insomnia with no side effects. I will give credit to the clinic I attended for recommending behavior modification. I take full responsibility for not believing in or pursuing behavior modification on my own or with the aid of my referring physician. I give the clinic two thumbs down for not offering a program through their clinic. Additionally, I give them two more thumbs down (it is a shame that I don't have more than two hands and two thumbs because I would turn them all down) as even today the clinic has no program for behavior modification and sleep hygiene, according to the receptionist. After completing the original draft of this paper, I did a lot of research on the Internet finding that there are many good sleep clinics that provide a total package of services. The methods I use to treat my insomnia in this book are all practiced in some form or fashion by the better sleep clinics. I cannot take credit for being so smart that I developed these ideas. All I did was put a package of good ideas together and make them work for me.

I firmly believe that a great number of you can eliminate your insomnia by following the steps that worked for me. It is a matter of conviction and dedication to ending the nightly ordeal that is ruining your life. There are many reasons for insomnia. You may have some unrealized condition that is preventing you from sleeping, or you might just need the support of a clinic to be successful with behavior modification. If you can't do it on your own, I hope at least this book will somehow convince you that you can improve your sleep without medication and that behavior modification techniques can work for you. Look for a good sleep disorders clinic by questioning others that have gone through a program. The American Sleep Disorders Association is a professional sleep organization that can provide you with a state-by-state list of their accredited sleep clinics. You can access this information at their web site, http://www.asda.org/centers.htm or you can write to:

American Sleep Disorders Association
1610 14th Street NW
Suite 300
Rochester, MN 55901

Don't be afraid to ask the clinic questions: "Do you offer behavior modification programs?" "Do you provide ongoing support while I am relearning my sleep habits?" "Will you provide referrals of people who have received alternate forms of treatment?" Finding a good sleep clinic should be no different from finding a good doctor or electrician or baby-sitter. If you do not feel comfortable with the sleep clinic in your vicinity, consider looking in another town. This is your life. Any time and money spent for a better quality of life pales in comparison to the benefits that you would derive from going through a successful program.

Subject: Trazodone and Ambien
From: Jennifer *
Date: Wed, Mar 11, 1998 19:13 EST
Message-id: *

I have insomnia, and I've finally managed to get a message through to my doctor explaining that I want to see a sleep specialist. I've been on Ambien for over a year. I'm frustrated, because my doc, without bothering to ask me any questions or actually talking to me, decided to try Trazodone in place of the Ambien. First, I've already tried Trazodone - probably two years ago now, maybe a little less. It wasn't effective, and to get me to sleep we had to up the dosage to the point where the skin on my hands started coming off. (one of the side effects)
Second, pulling someone off Ambien abruptly is not a good idea. It's a physically addictive drug.
But being a good sport, I went ahead and tried it last night. After only half an hour, I could barely breathe through my

nose. It wasn't like a cold or allergies, it was more like a wall had been put up at the top of my nose with just a tiiiny hole so that if I concentrated and breathed very slowly I could sneak some air through. It was worse laying down than when I was sitting up. I was also extremely disoriented and dizzy, so I couldn't really get out of bed and find something else to do while I waited to breathe again. It was five hours before I could go to sleep. It's now been about fifteen hours since I took the Trazodone (50mg) and I am still extremely mentally impaired - disoriented, dizzy, fuzzy-headed. (So I am hoping this post makes sense!)

Now they're trying to decide what to do with me next. I'm not sure what to do, either. Do I go along for a little while, and prove to the doc that the solution isn't to drug me into a stupor? Or do I attempt to pay for a sleep specialist on my own? (My insurance won't cover anything that is not a referral from my doctor)

Sorry this turned out to be so long!

Jen

Subject: Re: ISO insomnia help
From: *
Date: 1997/09/27
Message-ID: *

I keep reading in this newsgroup about seeing a good sleep specialist for help with insomnia. I've had insomnia for roughly 16 years. My doctor sent me to a sleep "specialist", and the specialist decided that insomnia was my "thing" .Just like some people have back troubles, heart problems, etc., my weakness was the inability to sleep. She felt it was due to my personality (I had suggested that's what I thought the problem was, and she agreed); I tend to think a lot, worry over minor disturbances, for example, and cannot seem to block out thoughts (not always negative) from my mind at bedtime.

If anyone knows of a good sleep specialist in the Halifax, Nova Scotia area, would you please e-mail me. I had resolved to just put up with my problem, even though I know the quality of my life is not what it should be.

However, after reading some of the articles in this newsgroup, it sounds to me like I should not give up quite so easily.
Thanks.

Subject: Re: Trazodone and Ambien
From: *
Date: Wed, Mar 11, 1998 20:28 EST
Message-id: *

* wrote:

Having tried the GP route myself, I can vouch for the fact that only a specialist knows enough about sleep problems to help. I was fortunate that my insurance didn't require a direct referral. However, you might want to check your policy carefully. See if the policy has a separate provision for mental health that doesn't require a referral from a GP. Many policies have separate procedures set up for this. If it does, you may be able to find a psychiatrist that specializes in sleep problems. In my case, while the listing was under a psychiatrist, the person I actually saw was a psychologist who was also a phsycian's assistant. My insurance paid without a second thought.

Also, if your doctor won't refer you, there is usually some procedure by the provider to allow you to either get another opinion or appeal directly to the insurance company. Unfortunately, this may require sorting through the language of the policy. If your insurance carrier has a person who's job it is to help you sort through the policy, call that person.

Good luck.

Last Word on Medications

I still take issue with the use of prescription medications for insomnia. I do feel as though the responsible sleep specialist will not use sleeping pills for other than a short term solution to get you through a tough period. I still see the liberal use of prescription medications for restless legs syndrome. Medications do provide relief for some from the symptoms of RLS but usually do not eliminate the condition. Furthermore, some medications, despite helping the patient sleep, have a side effect of making the condition worse during the day when it had previously not been a problem. Weigh the results of taking medication with side effects against alternative forms of treatment. Remember, I have had restless legs syndrome and continue to do so to a certain degree. I do not pretend to have symptoms nearly as bad as some other sufferers that I have read about. But I was diagnosed with "periodic movement of sleep" and was prescribed Klonopin, which I never took. I may even still have the leg movements. I do know that I am sleeping better than I have in years. My restless legs do not seem to be as bad as they were prior to my "cure". If I still have "periodic movement of sleep," it doesn't really bother me. Sure, I still have days when I feel more tired than normal, even though I felt I got a great night's sleep the night before. Maybe my legs moved and affected the quality of my sleep. Well, not everything in life is perfect. My body seems to do much better without the use of medications.

Am I suggesting that you not take medications? Absolutely not. You and your doctor should make rational decisions weighing the pros and cons of the medication and consider the potential side effects and possible tolerance. Read what the drug manufacturer has to say about the use of its medication for sleep. I am not aware of any manufacturer saying its medication will eliminate the problem for anything other than a short period of time. If something else such as behavior modification can work, give it a shot. You may not get that instant drug induced feeling, but if behavior modification works, you do not have to worry about dependence, withdrawal, side effects, and the correct dosage. As I discussed earlier, the term tolerance means that over time your body counters the effects of the medication you are taking. Every person responds differently. Just remember, with the correct behavior modification, each new day can bring better consequences, while each new day of taking a drug results in more tolerance against the drug.

Trazodone, Bad reaction? HELP!!!

Posted by * on March 07, 1998 at 08:34:29:

I was prescribed Trazodone well over a year ago to off set the side effects(insomnia) of the anti-depressant I am using(effexor). Started to experience problems in the last 2 mths. I was using 1/4-1/2 of 50mg. when I needed it. Then before Christmas, Started having to take a whole pill to get any effect. Also previously, it would only take 20-30 mins to fall asleep. Now it takes 2-3 hours, and then I only sleep 2-3 hours. AND I am sleepy all day.

I suspected I might have developed a tolerance, or an adverse reaction, as I have had this problem before with other drugs or herbal remidies (I had a terrible reaction to Valerian!) So two days ago, I threw out the last of my script. Now I get to sleep around 4:00 a.m. Wake up after 2-3 hours. During the day I am still sleepy, and will get to the point where I cannot stay awake. But then again, If I nap, I will only sleep an hour or so.

So, I am trying not to nap, avoiding sugar, caffine, etc. I am hoping that eventually I'll return to normal. I have had insomnia, on and off for years, but have attributed it to stress, as I can sleep at times.
Although I have always woken up in the night.

Sorry this is soooo long! I get carried away. Any suggestions would be appreciated.

Thanks, *

Subject: PLMD and RLS my story
From: gthorpe@netspace.net.au (Gary Thorpe)
Date: Wed, Apr 15, 1998 00:21 EDT

Just another stich in the tapestry

In March 1997 I was diagnosed with Periodic Limb
Movement Disorder at the Epworth Sleep Disorders Unit here
in Melbourne Australia.

Great little exersize all wire up and nowhere to go.

The "Cure" was the problem, 500ugm Clonazepam for the
rest of your life, going on and off it so as to not reduce its
effect. It eventually ceased having any effect so I was then
put on 100mg of Carbamazepine it has worked, though is the
zonked out day after really worth it. Anyway who wants to be
pill poping forever.
With that in mind I thought a try down the alternate medicine
path would be the go, so off to the Chinese Herbalist.
What an experience, the pile of compost that I had to brew
for a week and drink twice a day was to say the least a case of
the cure being worse than the desease, apart from the stench
you would have to be super human not to puke drinking the
stuff. Needless to say this treatment path was soon
abandoned. Next was the another natural cure, good old
Valerian, again only mixed success was acheived.
Almost all hope had evaporated when I remembered an
article about RLS documenting a study conducted by
Christopher Early, MD, PhD, from the Sleep Disorders
Center at The Johns Hopkins University of Medicine, where
when comenting on the Dopaminergic Dilemma, 25% of all
patients stopped all medication, instead relying on
alternatives such as BICYCLING BEFORE BEDTIME
Well how about that, I gave 10 minutes a night a try and
guess what, No More PLMD or RLS, and with the presence
of hindsite my problems really only became evident after I
had stopped riding my bike to work.

I hope this experience might help someone else, if it helps
just one other person then the post was worth it

Gary Thorpe
      gthorpe@netspace.net.au

I really hesitated before using the following post. When it was posted on the Internet, quite a few of the respondents took offense to the content, perhaps thinking the author was trivializing the treatment of sleep problems. I personally think that at least numbers 1-5 are compatible with the suggestions in this book. Also, I have no problem with number 6.

Subject: uplift. up and up
From: Francis Michael Smith <me11@soas.ac.uk>
Date: Wed, Mar 25, 1998 18:14 EST
Message-id: *

Dear Sleep Disorder Group,

I enjoyed reading the stories here on the newsgroup about sleep disorders.

I had terrible trouble sleeping and was usually exhausted.

I overcame it in a week much to my great relief with the following regime

(1) Eating vegetarian and wholemeal food only *(Quit cheese. milk, redmeats esp.)
(2) Not eating after 8pm except fruit
(3) Deep breathing(Diaphramatic) 2x a day
(4) Relaxation Techniques
(5) Eating fruit for breakfast (Freshly juiced at home)
(6) Swim or make love each day

Part IV

RESULTS

The following section will show you what is possible if you embark on a journey to end your insomnia. There is nothing here that you cannot achieve for yourself.

CHAPTER THIRTEEN

My Results...It Can Happen to You

When I began my "cure", my best guestimate was that I needed six hours of sleep to be functional each day. (I wasn't even sure about the six hours. Anytime I slept that long I usually had trouble getting to sleep the next night, so I figured six hours might be oversleeping). My sleep had been so erratic that it was really hard to guess, but I knew if I slept six hours that I could perform well the next day. Prior to my "cure", I had been waking up most mornings between 8:00 and 8:30. (On several occasions I had slept even later when I was not getting to sleep until 5:00 or 6:00 in the morning). This schedule was fine, as I worked out of my house starting around 9:00 a.m. each day.

I decided not to be too extreme in changing my wake-up time, so I chose 7:30 a.m. For me that would be something of a push. *Do not make too radical of a change to your current times. If you are currently getting up at 8:00 and ultimately want to start waking at 6:00, designate 7:00 or 7:30 as your initial target.* Accordingly, my bedtime was set for 1:30. Although I was seldom sleeping by that time, I was a little concerned about the late hour. I had almost always tried to be in bed quite a bit earlier than 1:30, even though I seldom stayed there. I was also concerned since I was in the middle of one of my bad sleep cycles. I had only been getting a couple of hours of very poor quality sleep every night, and I was exhausted. I was afraid that adjusting my hours would make matters even worse. Of course, it was because this last cycle was so bad that I decided a change had to be made. I refused to continue living my life like that.

I spent the first night of my "cure" reading one of my old books on insomnia. Usually these books would help me sleep. One, they were boring and, two, they usually made me relax and not worry quite as much about insomnia ruining my health. Around 12:30 I was still not very sleepy, but I did finally go to sleep some time around 2:30 (when you are keeping your sleep diary, you have to use your best guess sometimes). Although I really didn't want to, I did get up at 7:30 a.m. I felt pretty tired. Even more importantly, this was the first time in quite a while that I had gotten up at a set time. I realized at this point that I had developed a bad habit of letting myself sleep in. It would take a while to get used to waking at a set time. In any event, once I got over the initial drowsiness, I actually had a pretty good day. Remember, I had slept about five hours the night before, which was much better than normal.

The second night I was prepared to stay up until 1:30. I found out something amazing that first night. I could not stay awake. I kept dozing on the couch. I did everything in the world to stay awake, but I kept dozing. *Remember, the pressure to go to sleep has been removed.* Finally at 12:30, I decided I couldn't take it any more and went to sleep. Immediately. I only woke and got out of bed twice. I did snack both times. I got up at 7:30 a.m. as scheduled and really felt great.

What I discovered in the first few weeks was that the system worked! However, any time I cheated, I usually paid for it either by having problems going to sleep or staying asleep the next night. Most of the time when I stayed up until my designated time like I was supposed to, I would have to struggle to stay awake the next night. *What a great new problem, fighting to stay awake until bedtime! Who would have ever believed this? I was getting decent sleep night after night and feeling better during the day than I had in years!* Every day that I experienced positive results, I found myself becoming more and more excited. I will tell you right now that the more you stick to the program, the better your results will be. *This program works!*

I used the first couple of weeks to refine my sleep habits and my pre-sleep routine. I also used the time to develop the deep breathing and relaxation techniques, as well as methods to free my mind of obsessive thoughts. I hit a disappointing stretch where I was awake three nights in a row until 3:30, but that just emphasized the progress I had made. Before I started my treatment my very best nights were getting to sleep about 3-3:30. *If I had slept four straight hours for three consecutive nights, I would have been tickled to death.* Now in a matter of a couple of weeks, getting only this much sleep was a disappointment. The "cure" was working, even though there were a couple of minor setbacks. Furthermore, by keeping my sleep diary daily, I was able to pinpoint those factors that caused me to stay awake longer on those nights, such as a late bedtime snack. The three disappointing nights made me realize the importance of my pre-sleep routine. I needed the time before I settled in for sleep to rid my body and mind of any distractions. No matter how late I stayed out or how late I worked, I learned to lay on the couch and relax prior to bedtime, even if I felt I could go straight to bed. Also, I learned the importance of staying with my designated times.

One Night of Insomnia (Seven Weeks Later)

Over the last seven weeks, in addition to the occasional bad nights where I was up until 3:30, I have had one night where I did not get to sleep until 6:00 am. I still got up at 7:30, just like the plan calls for, even though it was a weekend. Although I have had a few bad nights, I am absolutely thrilled, as I haven't slept this well in years. I will say that the day after being awake until 6:00 was exactly as promised, tough but manageable. Your past experience with complete fatigue has come as a result of night after night of insomnia. Now you are solving your problem, and, even if you have a bad night here and there, you will function just fine. The day after I slept only an hour and a half, I still was able to exercise vigorously for one and one half hours, fill in as coach for my youngest son's basketball team, and work in the yard raking leaves as planned for three hours that afternoon. All without yelling at anyone. As a matter of fact, I was pretty happy. I discovered one bad night did not make me feel wasted like I thought it might. Was I tired? Yes. I was much more tired than normal, a fact I discovered, especially once I slowed down. I think it is better to stay even more active on a day following marginal sleep to keep the adrenaline flowing. I was able to stay awake until my designated time that night (it wasn't easy), and I slept great the next night and the next. I have not had another bad night like that since. *So remember, if you do happen to have a bad night every once and a while, do not worry! The next day will be tolerable.* What will be intolerable is if you quit doing or start cheating on the things that will end your insomnia. *You are now in control.*

Ten Weeks Later

I am writing this section ten weeks into my "cure". I would like to characterize my current sleep as follows: I am getting seven and one-half hours of sleep most nights. I would say on an average that I fall asleep five nights out of seven within ten minutes of lying down, usually somewhere around 11-12:30. If I do go down at 11:00, I try to get up no later than 6:30 a.m. I usually wake up no more than once or twice a night. Rarely do I get out of bed when I awaken any more. It was not that hard to break the habit of getting out of bed every time I awakened, even for someone like me that used to snack so much during the night. I will still get a snack during the night, but only once or twice a week, as opposed to once or twice a night previously.

On the other couple of nights during the week, I will have to go back to the couch after fifteen to twenty minutes of trying to fall asleep. I really have to watch the urge to stay in bed rather than getting up when I can't fall asleep. I think this is probably another of the lazy habits I have developed over the years. When I do remain in bed, I rarely, if ever, fall asleep. It is much more effective to get up. Most of the time I will read or watch TV and get sleepy enough to return to bed within thirty minutes. I will have an occasional night where I am up until 2-3:30 a.m. I have had one additional night when I was awake until 6:00 a.m. That makes two bad nights of insomnia in the last ten weeks, as opposed to three and four nights a week prior to starting my cure. This additional bad night occurred several nights ago, and my sleep has been great ever since. I still keep my sleep diary every day, and on those rare occasions when I do have a problem, I can usually pinpoint the reason for not falling or staying asleep. If you are a chronic insomniac, I would recommend keeping your sleep diary for an extended period of time to reinforce your new habits.

I have found that stress and anxiety rarely, if ever, keep me awake as badly as they use to due to the steps I have incorporated into my "cure". My biggest problem is still cutting out the late night snacks. There is absolutely no doubt that the steps I have taken are responsible for the dramatic improvement in my sleep. My wife is telling everyone that the man she married has returned for the first time in a long time.

Fourteen Weeks Later

I cannot stress enough the importance of continuing your sleep diary daily to help you examine what your sleep was like the night before and why. Even with the great success I have had, I still have to continue tweaking things so I do not fall back into a pattern of insomnia again. I almost look at myself like a recovering alcoholic in that if I fall back into old habits, I will end up back where I started before my "cure". As I really don't have a support group to fall back on, my sleep diary serves as my substitute.

Recently I hit a streak where I had several pretty bad nights in a row. Instead of going to sleep at or near my designated time, I had to stay up until 3:00 for three straight nights. I was disappointed but used my diary to help make some changes. First of all, I cut my time in bed back to six and a half hours. I did fine with seven and a half hours for a while, but I noticed I was waking up more during the night. And when I awakened, I found it harder to ignore the urge to get up and snack and started going back to my old routine of middle of the night snacking. Since cutting my time back to six and a half hours, I get to sleep much easier again, and I do not wake up as often.

The second adjustment I made had to do with my pre-sleep routine. I found on those nights when I did not feel quite so sleepy and might otherwise end up staying awake until 3:00 or so that I did much better reading than just watching television. Reading just seems to take my mind off of everything else better than watching TV. During the three consecutive bad nights I had recently, I was having a problem getting very sleepy at bedtime. *Some very unpleasant memories came back to me of lying on the couch until the wee hours of the morning.* When I started reading again, especially on those nights I suspected I might have trouble falling asleep, I found myself getting so drowsy that sleep came easily again. I had gotten lazier. It is easier to lie on the couch and watch television than it is to pull out a book and read it. Although I do not read every night, I will read on those nights that it seems I am a little more keyed up. *Don't get lazy and make the same mistakes I did. Constantly experiment with changes if you see a problem developing.*

The main point I want to make here is for you not to get complacent. After some early success, do not go back to your old habits. The changes you have made were not that hard. By keeping a daily diary, it is much easier to spot those things that you let sneak back into your life that can start negatively affecting your sleep. Remember, you have taken charge of your life once again. Keep the momentum going.

Eighteen Weeks Later

At the end of the "Fourteen Week Later" section, I said I almost felt like a recovering alcoholic. I now know that I have to be careful, or I can "fall off the wagon". I am so convinced that this is true that I now consider myself a "recovering insomniac". I know that any time I cheat on the program, I have to pay the price. I will have trouble falling asleep, waking up, or getting back to sleep.

It was during this period that I read <u>Sleep Thief</u>, a book about restless legs syndrome that I mentioned earlier in my text. Coincidentally(?), I experienced symptoms of restless legs for five straight days after reading the book. I had experienced fewer noticeable symptoms of restless legs since I started this program. Did reading the book have something to do with the reappearance of the symptoms? I doubt it, but who knows? There was one very positive experience as a result of this bout with restless legs. This is the time I finally discovered the benefits of a hot bath as related earlier in the text. The symptoms of my restless legs usually abated. Even more importantly, I learned how relaxing a hot bath could be and started incorporating it into my sleep routine.

I have now changed to six hours and forty-five minutes a night (11:45-6:30) for my Designated Amount of Time in Bed. I still have nights when I might not fall asleep immediately and have to return to my pre-sleep ritual. I still have nights when I awaken after an hour of sleep and have to return to the couch. And, every once in a while, I will still be awake until three in the morning. The most important thing that I have learned is that I rarely am exhausted the next day. An occasional bad night is an inconvenience, but there is no cumulative fatigue like that experienced when I had night after night of insomnia. I don't worry about the bad nights because I have learned that this plan works, and I know I will soon return to normal.

My blood pressure now runs about 115/74 the first thing in the morning and my pulse rate in the 60's. Last week my pulse rate in the middle of the day was running in the 50's. I actually was concerned about it. If you remember before I cured my insomnia, my pulse rate would run about 90 in the middle of the day, even when I was resting. Today my blood pressure in the middle of the day was 105/74—WOW!

CHAPTER FOURTEEN

Summary

I want to restate those things that will help eliminate your insomnia.

1. Prepare a sleep biography recalling all of those events that have led to the bad sleep habits you have formed. By looking the problem directly in the eye, you will realize the silly habits you have developed and how you can change them by following the plan.

2. Realize that <u>you</u> are the only answer to your sleep problem. You are the one that got yourself into the mess you are in now. And remember, insomnia is a non-addictive habit that can be easily broken.

3. Start a nightly sleep diary which will help you identify those daily circumstances that have an impact on your sleep. Experiment with changes such as the amount of sleep you need each night, the time you go to bed, amount of caffeine you consume each day, the time that you exercise, etc. to see how each affects your sleep. Also, be aware of any stressors that disrupt your sleep.

4. Develop a nightly pre-sleep routine. Use this as a transition period between your daily activities and your nightly slumber. Let your stress ooze out before lying down for the night.

5. Do not go to sleep until your designated time. You do not want to spend unnecessary and damaging time in the bedroom. If you must go to sleep earlier, cut your time in bed correspondingly, waking up at an earlier time (see "Adjustments" above).
6. Develop deep breathing and muscle relaxation techniques for use when you lie down as your final step before sleep. Also develop a method to rid your mind of obsessive thoughts.
7. Never sleep past your Designated Wake-Up Time, even on weekends. No exceptions! Even if you sleep little or none the night before.
8. Be committed. If you want to end your insomnia problems once and for all, be dedicated to this plan.

Always Remember:

Only you can change your sleep habits. Do not look for the answer in a medicine bottle. If you take sleeping pills, use them only for temporary relief. If you are concerned that you have become dependent on your sleeping pills, have you doctor help you break the addiction.

Do not worry about missing sleep occasionally. You will be able to function more than adequately the next day.

Do not try to bully sleep; it must come naturally. Follow the steps in this book, and it will.

If you are not close to sleep fifteen to twenty minutes after lying in bed, go to another room and engage in another activity such as reading or watching television.

Make adjustments wisely. Make sure you are ready for the adjustment.

Cut down on your caffeine intake, particularly in the evening. Remember chocolate contains caffeine.

Try not to eat dinner or heavy snacks too late in the evening. Eat a well-balanced diet. If you have problems with bingeing, examine the foods you are eating now and cut out those that are triggering your cravings. Monitor your use of sugar and artificial sweeteners to see if they impact your ability to sleep well.

Try to stop smoking. Tobacco is a stimulant.

Do not use alcohol to go to sleep. It may help you to sleep, but your quality of sleep will not be as good.

Develop a good exercise routine. Regular exercise will assist you in developing an overall better lifestyle and will aid in the production of serotonin. The production of serotonin will help improve your mood, eliminate your insomnia, and curb your cravings for food.

Take the steps necessary to reduce the controllable stressors in your life which interfere with your ability to relax. No success is worth the loss of family or friends, and it is certainly not worth an early grave. Take some time to do the things that you enjoy.

Keep a positive outlook on this program as well as life in general. Remember, positive thoughts bring positive results. Don't let a negative outlook spoil your enjoyment of life. But most importantly ... Start Living Again!

> *We are committing an unspeakable crime against ourselves when we drown ourselves in negative thinking.*-Maxie Dunham

> *Believe you can, and you can!*-Dr. Norman Vincent Peale

As you and I both have discovered, chronic insomnia has a tremendous impact on your overall quality of life. If you are like me, you may have withdrawn somewhat from a healthy overall lifestyle. You will now feel better than you ever thought you would again. No more daily worry about whether or not you will sleep again. You will find yourself rediscovering your energy supply. You will quit being so grumpy all of the time. You will now have the confidence to go after that promotion, or to pursue the other job offer, or take on a second job. Life is great! You are once again a living, breathing, normal participant. You will now feel like becoming a part of society once again. You won't have to worry about whether or not to accept an invitation to a social event or if you should become an officer in the parent-teachers club. But the most important thing that you need to do is to show your family that the normal, loving, caring member is back with them. Life is wonderful!

When you have problems in life, they can be self-perpetuating. You can't sleep. You are frustrated. Your quality of work suffers. You miss the big promotion. You suffer financially as a result. You become more and more depressed. The depression makes your insomnia worse. Your insomnia makes your day-to-day performance and your depression worse. Round and round it goes.

Well, everything is now going to change. Don't sit around and anticipate the worst. This insomnia plan is absolutely going to work for you. Get out and enjoy life again. Join a club. Travel. Coach your son's Little League team. Start regular exercise again. Have friends over to your house. They use to enjoy coming as much as you enjoyed having them. Take your spouse out to dinner. Take your family to the zoo. Play out in the yard with your children. Live! Love! Join! Volunteer! Help others! Be a real member of the human race! And when you do, and if you see me on the street, tell me, "thanks". Because, if I know I helped you, I know that I have once again become a functioning part of the human race also. I had almost given up on that hope.

> *Blessed is the person who is too busy to worry in the daytime and too sleepy to worry at night.*-Unknown

Good Luck! You are taking the steps necessary to reclaim your life.

> *Expect the best and get it!*-Unknown

CHAPTER FIFTEEN

Feedback

As I told you in "A Note to Readers" at the start of this book, I sent the book to several friends, doctors, and insomniacs to get feedback. I offered the manuscript on the Internet so that I could get feedback from insomnia sufferers whom I had never met. I felt this would provide me with additional comments that were not influenced by a personal relationship. I received e-mail from Hong Kong, Australia, and Canada in addition to the U.S. I think you should find some comfort in the fact that insomnia is an equal opportunity malady.

Many changes to the initial draft of this book were made as a result of comments and suggestions sent to me by these readers. I thank all of you that contributed for your input. Your positive comments also gave me the encouragement to make the necessary changes and finish the book. I learned there were several concepts in the original draft that I did not adequately explain. I was pleased to learn that the book motivated some insomniacs to use behavior modification rather than drugs as a possible solution for their sleep problem. As I mentioned in the "Note to Readers" at the start of the book, I was absolutely amazed that the readers of my first draft were so intrigued by my personal quest to cure my insomnia. One respondent told me she cried because she had had many of the same experiences. She had always been terribly embarrassed by the fact that she stayed in bed every morning to catch up on her sleep while her husband got their children off to school each day. Several respondents had gone through progressions similar to mine with their insomnia, finding no relief from sleeping pills or alcohol.

Some, like me, had quit trying to cure their insomnia with pills and alcohol when they realized their condition was not improving. They seemed to embrace the concept of the plan very well. It was very disturbing for me to hear from those who were absolutely terrified to stop taking their medication, herbs, or alcohol. These were many times the same people who made the strongest pleas for help. They fully realized the ineffectiveness of what they were currently trying. They were getting little or no sleep. Some even acknowledged that their insomnia was worse than before the advent of taking the drug (or drugs). They were constantly changing their medication, seeking the perfect sleeping pill. The following is not a quote but rather a compilation of several responses to me from people who would not or could not quit their medication or alcohol:

> "I became more and more anxious as the evening went along. About 1:30, I became afraid so I took a sleeping pill (or antidepressant or both) to help me relax. I still didn't get over an hour's sleep. I desperately need to get some sleep tonight. I can't go on this way. I have set up another appointment with my doctor, and we are going to try another medication in conjunction with what I am already taking. I feel certain your plan will work, but now is not the best time for me to try it. When I get things straightened out a little more, I will try again."

The sad thing is that this was the first night they tried the program, and they had already given up. I can only pray for these people. The sleeping pill, no matter how ineffective and destructive it may be, is a crutch these users cannot put away. "Help me. I am willing to try anything."—as long as it is a pill or herb or alcohol. If this describes your condition, and you don't think you can make the change necessary to get your life back in order, see a qualified sleep specialist. If you are just starting to experiment with the use of sleeping aids, be aware of what can potentially happen to you. On the bright side, I have had people respond very positively saying the book gave them the motivation to get with their doctor and stop taking their sleeping pills.

I would like to leave you with a comment written to me by a gentleman from Hong Kong reprinted directly from his e-mail:

> "I do not think it is proper to describe insomnia as a monster. You must ask a superman to crush a monster. But insomnia can never be conquered by any means. It can only be appeased like a cat. Whenever I find hard to fall asleep, I just tell my cat calmly, "Well, baby you don't want to sleep? Let's enjoy this book together". Nine out of ten times my cat will soon beg me to close the book and in 5 minutes I fall asleep soundly after switching off my lamp."

Afterword

I am writing this particular section on March 22, 1998, some twenty-two weeks into my "cure". I finally let someone at a sleep clinic read my draft knowing that I had stepped on a lot of toes in this field. Here is the response in part that I received by e-mail from Julia Thomas. She is with the Insomnia Clinic of the Methodist Hospital Sleep Disorders Center which is run by a University of Memphis student psychologist with Dr. Kenneth Lichstein as the supervising Clinical Psychologist:

> "I have finished your manuscript, at this point. Overall, I thought it was very good. You mentioned near the end, the importance of having support. Your book provides a pseudo support group to insomnia sufferers. The great value of support groups are being realized in a variety of fields from Narcotics Anonymous, to Domestic Violence victims, to a variety of cancer support groups (I am currently co-facilitating a breast cancer support group). I would recommend your book to clients/patients etc. for this reason........
>
> ......One thing that stands out at me as disturbing is your attitude towards psychologists, and I will assume other mental health professionals. I was hoping that like other issues (e.g. relaxation methods) you were initially against, that you would change your perspective at the end. I was sad to not see this. I am afraid, as I have noticed in others, that you are not aware of what mental health professionals (MHPs) do in 1998. You seem a knowledgeable individual. Have you ever been to a MHP? From your writing, it does not appear that you are aware that MHP's, among other things, provide exactly what you were seeking—help with

your insomnia via behavioral modifications. I am a student psychologist. My emphasis is in behavioral medicine. That means I will be working with "normal" individuals in a medical hospital (not a psychiatric hospital or wing) to help them cope/deal with their medical condition, as well as their psychological/emotional/cognitive condition. It's kind of like when you rightly say, depression can cause insomnia, but just because you have insomnia does not mean that you're depressed—a psychologist can help psychopathology, but that does not exclude them from helping behaviorally related difficulties. Psychology is the study of human behavior. What contributes to human behavior? a countless variety of things.

I guess my plea to you is that you help the field of psychology and those who can benefit from our services by helping to inform your readers that although some MHPs still make use of a leather couch and analyze dreams and only psychotic people go to them, the mental health field long ago outgrew that stereotype. We are everywhere helping a wide variety of people (not just those who "have something wrong with them", namely in the head) for a great variety of reasons. Please, help people not fear stigmatization for going to a psychologist or other MHP. The field has grown tremendously, but somehow people don't know about it.

Congratulations, though, on writing this book. You should be proud of not only your end product, but also the process along the way."

Those words had a dramatic impact on me. I realized that I had an attitude like everyone else when I went to the sleep clinic. I, too, wanted some kind of miracle. The clinic did tell me behavior modification was one of the answers that I was seeking. I never pursued it. I blamed this on the fact that they did not offer a comprehensive program including behavior modification. I probably would have never participated anyway. That was not the answer I was looking for at the time. My questions are: Why are we so willing to take about any prescription medicine that our doctor gives us, most of the time without question, but we have such an aversion to accepting assistance from qualified mental health professionals? Is it pride or is it "I really don't want someone else telling me how to live my life" or "Will everyone think that there is something mentally wrong with me?"

As I was writing this book it occurred to me that it was going to be a "rah, rah" book to get others to realize that behavior modification techniques are what is needed to combat their insomnia. They didn't need pills. They didn't need herbs. The readers and I could do everything on our own. We didn't need anyone else. Well, you know what? I was lucky. It was just the right set of circumstances that allowed me to overcome my problem. If I had not read the books and articles by those that I have criticized in this book, I couldn't have done what I did. I still feel as though it is possible for many, if not most of you, to treat your insomnia and beat it just like I did without going to a sleep specialist or a sleep clinic. But I now say to you, if you can't do it on your own, you should go to an expert. Do your homework as to who will be the most qualified to help you beforehand, but go to a sleep specialist. How much money is your well-being worth to you? In my case it would have been worth much more than I was ever charged. Furthermore I say to you, let this book prove to you that non-medicinal techniques work. Trust your sleep specialist when he tells you behavior modification will help cure your insomnia.

The following letter from one of the readers of an early draft further emphasizes what was said above:

"John,

Just finished the book. It was great.

As you freely admitted, there is nothing new here necessarily, but it does put a very comprehensive plan together for conditioned insomnia, whereas other books sometimes skim over the topic.

You're quite wrong about lacking writing ability. This was well written, funny, compassionate, and uncluttered. I should know because, although you didn't know this, I'm a literary agent by profession..........

..........Your advice, although I've encountered it before, is certainly based on good research. I've tried much of it at one time or another, with varying results, but I lacked discipline to do it right, as you have done.

But you have inspired me to give it another try! And I am very excited. (So excited, I won't fall asleep tonight.)

I must say, too, that I have discovered exactly the same things about sleep and insomnia as you have. It's spooky how similar our sleep problems have been..........

..........Coincidentally, I have started this very same sleep reduction program through the Catholic Medical Ctr Sleep Center in New Hampshire, and I'm already keeping a sleep diary.

I'm hoping between your comprehensive program and that of the sleep center, I'll finally get some Zzzzs. We'll see.

Thanks, thanks, thanks for the time you put in with me on this, and the trouble you took mailing it to me. I appreciate that level of thoughtfulness tremendously.

A big pat on the back for your efforts with the book. It is extremely well done and deserves recognition.

Sweet dreams!

mm, ca"

Where Do We Go From Here????

You have finished the book and are committed to taking the steps necessary to regain control of your life. (Some of you may realize that your problems are really not that bad. You now know that you shouldn't worry about occasional sleeplessness.) You have ruled out sleep apnea and primary depression as the cause of your insomnia. You have made sure the current medications you are taking are not the cause. You now need to put your heart and soul into changing your sleep habits. You knew the answer all along lay within you alone. Now it is time to call upon your inner strength and to discover you have what it takes.

Hopefully you will see your sleep improve almost immediately, like I did. But it may take months before you see the results you desire. If at the end of this period you have not improved, and your sleep is ruining your life and your health, it is time to see a sleep professional. Some of you have never seen a sleep specialist, now is the time. Others will have seen a professional previously, now is the time for reevaluation ... in retrospect, was the advice sound? If so, see him for the support you need. If you feel the necessity, find a new sleep professional that can help you find the rest you deserve every night.

My thoughts are with you.

APPENDIX

SLEEP BIOGRAPHY GUIDE

Name_____   Date _____

Use the following (as well as my biography) as a guide to writing your sleep biography:

How long have you had sleep problems?
What are your first memories of sleep problems?
Did you walk in your sleep as a child?
Did you have good sleep habits in elementary school, high school, and college?

Can you pinpoint the time and cause of your first sleep related problems?
Can you plot how the sleep problems became more chronic?

What major events in your life created sleep related problems?
For how long did the related problem last?

What have you done or taken to help you sleep better over the years?
Did you have any success with anything? Were the results usually temporary?

Do you smoke? How much? Do you smoke at bedtime? Do you get up during the night to smoke? Do you plan to quit? Did you already quit? Did quitting help your sleep?

Do you consume too much caffeine? From coffee? How much? Cokes? Chocolate? Medications? How late do you usually have caffeine? Do you plan to cut back or quit?

How much and how often do you drink alcohol or take recreational drugs? Do you ever drink or take recreational drugs to sleep? Do you find yourself awakening during the night after their use? Do you drink too close to bedtime? Are you an alcoholic? If not, do you still drink too much?

How would you rate your personality type?
A. Always in a hurry, a perfectionist, reactionary
B. Middle of the road
C. Laid back; don't worry, be happy

What is your outlook on life?
A. Everything is wonderful, optimistic
B. Middle of the road
C. Can't seem to find happiness, negative

Describe Your Current Sleep (What goes on from bedtime until time to get up?)

Is your sleep consistent every night? If not, describe your various sleep cycles?

SLEEP BIOGRAPHY

Name _____   Date _____

SLEEP DIARY GUIDE

Date _____
Designated Bedtime _____   Designated Wake-Up Time _____
Designated Amount of Time in Bed _____

A. Sleep

How did you sleep last night?
Excellent _____   Good _____   Fair _____   Poor _____   Don't Ask _____

What time did you lie down? _____   If not your designated time, why? _____

Did you use relaxation and deep breathing techniques? _____
Were they effective? _____

How long did it take you to go to sleep? _____

Before falling soundly asleep, did you have to get out of bed? _____
For how long? _____

What did you do during this time?
Watch TV _____   Read book _____   Try to sleep on couch (or elsewhere) _____
   Eat _____   Other (Explain) _____

If you did not go to sleep quickly, what was on your mind?
Job _____   Family _____   Financial _____   Worry about sleep _____
Other _____

How did you try to eliminate the thoughts? _____

How many times did you get up during the night? _____

What did you do when you got up?
Drink water _____   Eat _____   Use the bathroom _____   Read _____
Watch TV _____   Other (Explain) _____

How long did it take to get back to sleep? _____

If you could not get back to sleep, what did you think about?
Job _____   Family _____   Financial _____   Worry about sleep _____
Other _____

How did you try to eliminate the thoughts? _____

B. Today

What time did you wake up this morning? _____
If not your designated time, why? _____

How did you feel upon awakening? _____

How refreshed did you feel today? _____

Did you feel the need to nap? _____

C. Yesterday Evening

In the last couple of hours before sleep did you:
Drink Alcohol _____   Smoke or Chew Tobacco _____   Have Caffeine _____
Have a Late Dinner or Snack _____   Argue _____   Worry (about what) _____
Exercise _____   Work _____   Have Restless Legs _____
Other (explain) _____

Were you anxious about going to sleep? _____

Did you follow a pre-sleep routine? _____

Did your legs feel restless? _____
What did you do to eliminate the problem? _____

Did you take any medication, prescription or non-prescription, to assist your sleep?_____

Could you have fallen asleep in another room, but not in bed? _____

D. Yesterday

What factors occurred yesterday that you feel affected your sleep?

Alcohol _____   Caffeine _____   Tobacco _____
Slept too late yesterday morning _____   On Medication _____
Daytime nap (what time and how long) _____
Poor quality sleep the night before _____   General anxiety _____
Anxiety related to falling asleep _____   Generally Depressed _____
Some disturbing event _____   Other stressors (list) _____

E. Tonight

What can be done to sleep better tonight? _____

SLEEP DIARY WORKSHEET

Name_____   Date _____

Current Hours

<u>Sunday</u> <u>Monday</u> <u>Tuesday</u> <u>Wednesday</u> <u>Thursday</u> <u>Friday</u> <u>Saturday</u>

Normal Bedtime
Normal Wake Up

Average Hours of Sleep per Night _____

New Hours

I.   Designated Amount of Time in Bed _____ (Initially, the same as the minimum number of hours of sleep required to feel rested the next day)

II. Designated Wake-Up Time _____ (Seven days a week)

III. Designated Bedtime _____ (Number of hours for designated sleep time prior to designated wake-up time)
Example: Six hours of designated sleep with a 7:30 wake-up time = 1:30

Do you have a nightly pre-sleep routine? _____
Describe it. (If you do not currently have a routine, fill this in when you have and include the date) _____

Factors Affecting Sleep

How do you rate your general mood at this time?
Upbeat _____   Moderate _____   Depressed _____

Are there major events in your life at this time that you feel are affecting your sleep (such as a job change, death of a friend or loved one, marital or family problems, move, health problems, financial crises, general depression and/or anxiety)?
List _____

List other factors that you feel are contributing to your current sleep problems (caffeine, tobacco, alcohol, recreational drugs, restless legs, medications, stress, physical pain, bad diet, no exercise, indigestion or other stomach problems) _____
_____

SLEEP DIARY SAMPLE DAILY LOG

Date __Oct. 20, 1997__
Designated Bedtime __12:30__   Designated Wake-Up Time ___7:30___
Designated Amount of Time in Bed _7 hours_

(Please note that these are the original times I set. At this point I am just in my second week of my cure and want to wait a few more days before making any adjustments)

cure continues to work very well. went to bed at 12:30. was very tired on the couch and had to walk around several times to keep from falling asleep. legs were restless, but discomfort finally went away. fell asleep immediately. only woke up twice during the night and only got out of bed once. refrained from eating anything while up and went right back to sleep both times. rhonda got me up at 7:30. did not particularly want to get out of bed, but once up did fine. had plenty of energy all day.

Date __Nov. 21, 1997__
Designated Bedtime __11:30__   Designated Wake-Up Time ___7:00___
Designated Amount of Time in Bed _7 ½ hours_

(Please note that I kept my log daily, but have skipped forward to a month later. I have moved my bedtime to 11:30 and wake-up time to 7:00, increasing my time in bed to 7½ hours. I did not make any adjustments from my original times until I had first slept well for a couple of weeks . I stayed with these times after I found that they did not adversely affect my quality of sleep. I did have one real bad night about a week ago when I was up until 4:30, but have had no problems since.)

went to bed at 11:15 after I did everything I could to stay awake and couldn't. pretty impressed as I was afraid the blowup I had with my main customer today might keep me from falling asleep tonight. it was still on my mind when I lay down for sleep, but the deep breathing and relaxation, along with my refusal to think about it, worked. only took about ten minutes to fall asleep. got up once and snacked. need to cut it out as this is three nights in a row that I allowed myself to snack. I did go right back to sleep. woke up at 6:45 and had a great day.

Date __Nov. 22, 1997__
Designated Bedtime __11:30__   Designated Wake-Up Time ___7:00___
Designated Amount of Time in Bed _7 ½ hours_

gave in and ate a couple pieces of cake and drank a glass of milk around 10:45. was not sleepy at 11:30, so stayed up until 12:30. still could not get to sleep, so got out of bed at 12:45 and went back to couch. still didn't feel sleepy, but tried again at 1:30 and, with deep breathing and relaxation, fell asleep within minutes. woke up 2 or 3 times and really wanted to snack, but held out and fell back to sleep pretty quickly. got up at 7:05 and felt more tired than normal. need to stop snacking late and during the night. every time I do my sleep is not as good.

SLEEP DIARY DAILY LOG

Date _____
Designated Bedtime _____   Designated Wake-Up Time _____
Designated Amount of Time in Bed _____

Date _____
Designated Bedtime _____   Designated Wake-Up Time _____
Designated Amount of Time in Bed _____

Date _____
Designated Bedtime _____   Designated Wake-Up Time _____
Designated Amount of Time in Bed _____

INTERNET RESOURCES GUIDE

The following Internet sites are provided to give you more information resources regarding sleep and sleep disorders. The act of placing a site on the list does not indicate any manner of endorsement from the author for information presented in the site or for any products sold from the site. Likewise, the inclusion of a site below does not indicate an endorsement for this book from that organization. This list does not even begin to list all of the sites available, but will provide a good starting place. If you do not see the information you desire in the following, you can probably find it through one of the sites listed. Most of the sites below will have links to other locations with sleep related information. Also, make good use of the search engines available to you through your Web browser and be creative with the word or words you search ... try sleep, sleep disorders, insomnia, the specific disorder you want, etc.

Although some of the sites below have already been mentioned in the body of the book, most are new including topics that were not discussed in the book such as narcolepsy, dreams, and children's sleeping problems. If a description has quotation marks, the information was picked up directly from the site or a spokesperson for the site.

John Wiedman's Personal Site
http://www.insomniacure.com

In the development stage at the time of this writing, this site is anticipated to include information on this book, links to sleep and sleep disorder sites, and, possibly, a discussion forum for insomnia sufferers ... perhaps featuring the sharing of successful suggestions for treating insomnia.

Discussion Groups, Forums, and Message Boards

SleepNet Sleep Forum
http://www.sleepnet.com/wwwboard/wwwboard.html

Has several excellent forums on different sleep disorders for the public and for professionals. Many of the posts in this book came from these forums.

Sleep/Wake Disorders Canada
http://www.delphi.com/swdc/

Thrive-AOL, go to KEYWORD, enter **thrive@health**, messages, **sleep disorders**

Better Health-AOL, go to KEYWORD, enter **Better Health,** sleep disorders, under "support", hit go

Online Psych-AOL, go to KEYWORD, enter **Online Psych**, hit message boards, then **dreams** or **sleep disorders** (*the message board at the time of this publication was very strong for narcolepsy, but not for other sleep disorders*).

Thrive Sleep Disorder Message Boards Online
http://www.thriveonline.com/cgi-bin/webx.cgi?14@^38289@.e e8b987

Night Terrors
http://www2.micro-net.com/~dwr/messboard/messboard.html

Food Addictions-AOL, go to KEYWORD, enter **a&r** (addiction and recovery), hit message boards, then food addictions-*this will put you with the message board for Kay Sheppard, Overeaters Anonymous, and others.*

Fibromyalgia
http://www.tidalweb.com/fms/fmsbbs/

Newsgroups

Deja News
http://www.dejanews.com/

Deja News is a free service that allows the user to search the archives of more than 50,000 discussion forums, including Usenet newsgroups such as alt.support.sleep-disorder listed below. And while the newsgroups only carry old listings until the space allocated is used, Deja News still provides access to the older information. Use Deja News like a search engine to find all of the posts on a given topic such as sleep, sleep disorders, sleep apnea, etc.

alt.support.sleep-disorder
The most active sleep disorder site of which I am aware. Many of the posts in this book came from this site.

alt.dreams

alt.dreams.lucid

alt.drugs.caffeine-*I don't particularly care for the newsgroup, but the "Frequently Asked Questions" has a good deal of information.*

alt.med.cfs-Chronic Fatigue Syndrome Information

alt.med.fibromyalgia-Fibromyalgia information

alt.support.narcolepsy-Narcolepsy support group.

Chats

Sleep/Wake Disorders Canada
http://www.delphi.com/swdc/

Thrive-AOL, go to keyword, **thrive@health**, chats, sleep disorders support groups, go to health chat room

Monday 9pm-11pm EST: go to health chat room, hit private chat, type in "sleepers lounge"
Tuesday 9pm-11pm EST: go to health chat room
Wednesday 9pm-11pm EST: go to health chat room, private chat, type in "sleepers lounge"

Sleep Disorder Sites
These sites include extensive information on all sleep disorders with links to other sleep disorder sites.

Sleepnet
http://www.sleepnet.com/

"SleepNet was started to help get the word about sleep disorders and sleep deprivation to the public. One of the goals of SleepNet is to link all the sleep information located on the Internet."

Sleep Forum-presented by SleepNet
http://www.sleepnet.com/wwwboard/wwwboard.html

National Heart, Lung, and Blood Institute (NHLBI) Sleep Disorders Information
http://www.nhlbi.nih.gov/nhlbi/sleep/sleep.htm

Information about sleep disorders as well as about research and education. Presented by the National Heart, Lung, and Blood Institute (NHLBI), a part of the Federal Government's National Institutes of Health.

National Sleep Foundation
http://www.sleepfoundation.org/

Excellent information. Also listed under Sleep Organizations.

The Simmons Company
http://www.simmonsco.com/sleep.info/

Includes a sleep test (listed in the sleep disorder test classification) and *information on sleep disorders as well as information on sleep stages and REM sleep.*

The Sleep Medicine Home Page
http://www.users.cloud9.net/~thorpy/

This site features an extensive listing of sleep related links to other sites.

"This home page lists resources regarding all aspects of sleep including, the physiology of sleep, clinical sleep medicine, sleep research, federal and state information, patient information, and business-related groups."

Sleep/Wake Disorders Canada
http://www.geocities.com/HotSprings/1837/index.html

A comprehensive site listing many sleep disorders with its own support forum and chat room.

"Sleep/Wake Disorders Canada is a national, self-help registered charity dedicated to helping the thousands of Canadians suffering from sleep/wake disorders. SWDC have chapters across the country which provide a face to face forum for meeting others with sleep disorders and also provide much needed information and support. It's members work to improve the quality of life, alertness, and productivity of persons with sleep/wake disorders.

SWDC has information brochures, articles, booklets and videos for educational purposes and publishes a quarterly newsletter *Good/Night Good/Day*. As well, they run an annual conference and hold group meetings. They are an invaluable resource for both physicians and the public.
SLEEP/WAKE DISORDERS CANADA (AFFECTIONS DU SOMMEIL/EVEIL CANADA)
3080 Yonge Street, Suite 5055, Toronto, Ontario M4N 3N1. Telephone: (416) 483-9654 and 1-800-387-9253 for calls outside of Toronto. FAX: (416) 483-7081"

The Sleep Well
http://www-leland.stanford.edu/%7Edement/

This site has it all...from links to other sites, information on sleep disorders, how to become a sleep activist, recommended books and publications, self-tests, dreams, and children's sleep disorders to sleep humor and much more.

Specific Sleep Related Topics

BEDDING

American Innerspring Manufacturers (AIM)
http://www.aiminfo.org/

"AIM stands for American Innerspring Manufacturers, a non profit association that provides information on healthful sleep and sleep surfaces. Through their support of numerous scientific studies and national surveys, AIM has educated a generation of American Consumers on how to get a good night's rest, as well as what to know and look for when it comes to choosing bedding."

The Better Sleep Council
http://www.bettersleep.org/index.html

Includes tips for a good night's sleep as well as information about mattresses.

"Established in 1978, the Better Sleep Council (BSC) is a non-profit organization supported by the mattress industry. The BSC is devoted to educating the public about the importance of sleep to good health and quality of life and about the value of the sleep system and sleep environment in pursuit of a good night's sleep."

Relax The Back Store
http://www.relaxtheback.com/html/bedsleep.html

Information pertaining to their sleep system, as well as information on stress reduction.

SELECT COMFORT® Home Page
http://www.comfort.com/

Information on their sleep system.

Tempur-Pedic Online
http://www.tempurpedic.com/sleep.html

Site includes information on their sleep system as well as sleep links.

CAFFEINE

Frequently Asked Questions about Coffee and Caffeine
http://daisy.uwaterloo.ca/~alopez-o/caffaq.html

Everything you ever wanted to know about caffeine including where you find it and how it affects your health.

CHILDREN'S SLEEP PROBLEMS

The National Enuresis Society (NES) *(Bedwetting)*
http://www.peds.umn.edu/Centers/NES/

Address may change as likely merging with the National Kidney Foundation this year.
"The National Enuresis Society (NES) is a not-for-profit organization of doctors, medical personnel, and other persons dedicated to building greater awareness and understanding of enuresis. By creating this awareness and understanding, the NES hopes to help improve both the treatment of enuresis and the quality of life for children with enuresis and their families."

Sudden Infant Death Syndrome and Other Infant Death (SIDS/OID) Information Web Site
http://sids-network.org/

"This site is the growing collaborative effort of individuals from across the United States and around the world. This sites offers up-to-date information as well as support for those who have been touched by the tragedy of SIDS/OID."

Things That Go Wrong in the Night
http://kidshealth.org/parent/healthy/sleep_disorder.html

Excellent information on infant and childhood sleep disorders

CHRONIC FATIGUE SYNDROME (See also Newsgroups)

CFS Home Page
http://www.cdc.gov/ncidod/diseases/cfs/cfshome.htm

Presented by the Centers for Disease Control and Prevention Atlanta, Georgia, USA

Chronic Fatigue Syndrome
http://www.ncf.carleton.ca/freenet/rootdir/menus/social.servic
es/cfseir/CFSEIR.HP.html

This site was written by Sandy Shaw who has suffered from CFS for years.

DELAYED SLEEP PHASE SYNDROME

Delayed Sleep Phase Syndrome:
http://www.geocities.com/HotSprings/1123/dsps.html

"Delayed sleep phase syndrome (DSPS) is a fairly common disorder of sleep timing. People with DSPS tend to fall asleep at very late times, and also have difficulty waking up in time for normal work, school, or social needs...This document was written and distributed to provide information for the general public about aspects of sleep and sleep disorders. It is not medical advice, and individuals with a suspected or diagnosed sleep disorder should consult with a physician for advice regarding their own treatment." *Presented by Su-Laine Yeo who suffers from DSPS.*

DREAMS (See also, Discussion Groups)

The Association for the Study of Dreams
http://www.asdreams.org/

A non-profit organization promoting dream research.

EXCESSIVE DAYTIME SLEEPINESS

EDS (Excessive Daytime Sleepiness) Information Site
http://www.daytimesleep.org/suffer1a.htm

This site assists you in determining the underlying cause of your daytime sleepiness.

FIBROMYALGIA (See also Newsgroups, also see Message Boards)

The Mystery of Fibromyalgia
http://www.columbia.net/consumer/datafile/fibro.html

An article by John Palopoli, M.D. on a web site sponsored by Columbia/HCA Healthcare Corporation.

Living with Fibromyalgia (FMS) and Chronic Myofascial Pain Syndrome (MPS) The Invisible Disease
http://www.tidalweb.com/fms/

INSOMNIA

Sealy Sleep Information Center
http://www.sealy.com/sleephlp.asp

Presented by the Sealy Corporation, the largest mattress manufacturer in North America.

Tips for Restful Sleep
http://www.ghc.org/health_info/self/seniors/zzz.html

Presented by Group Health Cooperative-the nations largest member-governed healthcare organization: Information on insomnia including suggested ways to improve sleep.

Sleep/Insomnia Program
http://www.iris-publishing.com

"Recognizing the huge numbers of people who suffer from sleep problems, this site has help for insomnia, curious insomnia cures, and sleep information resource links."

Presented by Sarah Richards, MS, LPC, CCMHC (541)752-4228

Shuteye Online
http://www.shuteye.com/

Sponsored by G. D. Searle and Co.-a good reference site that takes into account your individual problem and suggestions for overcoming it.

MELATONIN

Melatonin Use Strongly Discouraged
http://nytsyn.com/live/Depression/227_081496_200130_2090.html

An article that is actually not as one-sided as the title indicates it might be.

The Miracle of Melatonin: Fact, Fancy and Future
http://ci.mond.org/9617/961712.html

Another article with a little more balance.

NAPPING

The World Nap Organization (WNO)
http://www.bluemarble.net/~amyloo/wno.html

A fun and interesting site by a support group for nap taking.

NARCOLEPSY (See also Newsgroups)

Stanford University Center For Narcolepsy
http://www-med.stanford.edu/school/Psychiatry/narcolepsy/

CURE NARCOLEPSY NOW!
http://www.users.cloud9.net/~thorpy/narc.htm

Narcolepsy Network
http://www.websciences.org/narnet/

"Narcolepsy Network is a national, non-profit organization incorporated in 1986. Our members are people who have narcolepsy (or related sleep disorders), their families and friends, and professionals involved in treatment, research, and public education regarding narcolepsy."

NUTRITION

The American Dietetic Association
http://www.eatright.org

No fad diets here, just good nutrition with well balanced meals.

NIGHT TERRORS (See also Message Boards)

Night Terrors
http://www2.micro-net.com/~dwr/

Comprehensive site by a sufferer. Includes a message board.

RESTLESS LEGS SYNDROME

Restless Legs Syndrome Foundation
http://www.rls.org/

"The Restless Legs Syndrome Foundation is a nonprofit 501(c)(3) agency that provides information about RLS; helps develop support groups; supports research to find better treatments and, eventually, a definitive cure; educates physicians and patients about RLS; and publishes a quarterly newsletter known as NightWalkers."

SAD (SEASONAL AFFECTIVE DISORDER)

Seasonal Light/SAD Homepage
http://www.geocities.com/HotSprings/7061/sadhome.html#top

"This site deals exclusively with SAD (Seasonal Affective Disorder) and seasonal light. It covers book listings, articles, and information on membership organizations and light-box and other seasonal light device manufacturers. From here are links to most of the seasonal sites."

http://www.nyx.net/~lpuls/sadhome.html-*a text only version of the above site.*

SHIFTWORK

Circadian Technologies, Inc. (CTI)
http://www.shiftwork.com/

"Circadian Technologies, Inc. (CTI) provides research, consulting, training and information services. Since 1983, CTI has developed and applied proven, state-of-the-art methods and techniques for improving alertness, safety and job performance in continuous operations."

SLEEP ARTICLES

The Future of Sleep
http://www.wired.com/wired/4.12/reality_check.html

Four authorities give their opinions relating to the timetable for a cure for snoring, the introduction of a non addictive sleeping pill, the elimination of the need for sleep, and dream inducers.

How to Feel Well Rested on Too Little Sleep-*Redbook*
http://homearts.com/rb/health/04sleef1.htm

Tips by Tamara Eberlein on overcoming sleep deprivation

In praise of sleep—the best medicine
http://www.menninger.edu/tmc_artmnt_sleep.html

By Jon G. Allen, PhD-explains what happens when you sleep

SLEEP AIDS

Better Sleep
http://www.drshane.com/masterset2.htm

Two audio tapes and a sleep guide to help you "ease into sleep".
1-888-DRSHANE

SLEEP APNEA AND SNORING

The American Sleep Apnea Association (ASAA)
http://www.sleepapnea.org

"The American Sleep Apnea Association was founded in 1990 as a non-profit 501(c)(3) organization by persons with apnea and concerned health care providers and researchers. The ASAA's mission is simple:

The American Sleep Apnea Association is dedicated to reducing injury, disability, and death from sleep apnea and to enhancing the well-being of those affected by this common disorder. The ASAA promotes education and awareness, the ASAA A.W.A.K.E. Network of voluntary mutual support groups, research, and continuous improvement of care."

Childhood Snoring When Is It Serious?
http://www.mayohealth.org/ivi/mayo/9512/htm/snoring.htm

From Mayo Clinic

Kerrin Leon White, M.D.   A Physician with Severe Sleep Apnea
http://www.geocities.com/HotSprings/Spa/4752/

"PURPOSE: To share with fellow sleep apnea sufferers what I learn in reading literature on sleep research, and to learn as much as possible from fellow patients."

Phantom Sleep Resources TM
http://www.newtechpub.com/phantom /

This site is often referenced by those who suffer from sleep apnea. It includes a self-scoring quiz, information on the book, "Phantom of the Night", and an excellent FAQ listed below.

"Resources and information about sleep and sleep disorders including snoring and sleep apnea for the public, patients, and professionals."

http://www.newtechpub.com/phantom/faq/osa_faq.html

Frequently asked questions regarding sleep apnea and snoring

Quietsleep
http://www.quietsleep.com/

"Welcome to Quietsleep - the Web's most complete and reliable source of information on oral appliance therapy for snoring and obstructive sleep apnea."

Snoring: Not Funny, Not Hopeless
http://www.netdoor.com/entinfo/snoreaao.html

A brochure from the American Academy of Otolaryngology-Head and Neck Surgery.

STRESS

Quanta Dynamics, Inc.
http://www.quantadynamics.com/

"Find relief for overcoming stressed out days and sleepless nights … Quanta Dynamics, Inc. is a provider of innovative programs to help people reduce stress, renew energy and increase productivity."

Quanta offers the Gift of Sleep CD set and holds seminars on stress reduction, shift work, and insomnia.

Sleep Disorder Tests

Self Test
http://www.sleep-sdca.com/consumer.htm

Presented by the Sleep Disorder Centers of America.

Simmons Sleep Test
http://www.simmonsco.com/sleep.info/sleeptest.html

Presented by the Simmons Company, the mattress people

The Sleep Test
http://www.nshsleep.com/test.cfm

Presented by Northside Hospital Sleep Medicine Institute in GA.

Other Sleep Organizations

American Sleep Disorders Association (ASDA) (See Sleep Disorder Centers)
http://www.asda.org/centers.htm

"The American Sleep Disorders Association (ASDA) is a professional medical association representing practitioners of sleep medicine and sleep research. Sleep disorders medicine is a clinical specialty concerned with diagnosis and treatment of patients with disorders of sleep and daytime alertness."

The American Psychiatric Association
http://www.psych.org/main.html

The American Psychological Association (APA)
http://www.apa.org/

"The American Psychological Association (APA), in Washington, DC, is the largest scientific and professional organization representing psychology in the United States and is the world's largest association of psychologists. APA's membership includes more than 155,000 researchers, educators, clinicians, consultants, and students. Through its divisions in 50 subfields of psychology and affiliations with 59 state, territorial, and Canadian provincial associations, APA works to advance psychology as a science, as a profession, and as a means of promoting human welfare."

The American Psychological Society
http://psych.hanover.edu/APS/

National Sleep Foundation
http://www.sleepfoundation.org/

"The National Sleep Foundation is a nonprofit organization that promotes public understanding of sleep and sleep disorders and supports sleep-related education, research and advocacy to improve public health and safety. Established in 1990, the Foundation relies on corporate and individual donations, and partnerships with corporations and government, to fund its many educational and research programs."

Sleep Home Pages-World's Sleep Pages
http://bisleep.medsch.ucla.edu/

"The Brain Information Service (BIS) at UCLA provides a 'storefront' for Home Pages for any sleep organization, entity or activity that promotes the research or treatment of sleep and sleep-related disorders."

The World Federation of Sleep Research Societies (WFSRS)
http://bisleep.medsch.ucla.edu/wfsrs/description.html

"The World Federation of Sleep Research Societies (WFSRS) was founded in 1987. Its mission was and is to encourage international collaborations, facilitate the generation and dissemination of information, and increase public awareness of the importance of sleep research and the impact of sleep disorders. The WFSRS is a Federation of the following societies:

Australasian Sleep Association (ASA)
Canadian Sleep Society (CSS)
European Sleep Research Society (ESRS)
Japanese Society for Sleep Research (JSSR)
Latin American Sleep Society (LASS)
Sleep Research Society (United States) (SRS)

The Asian Sleep Research Society
http://bisleep.medsch.ucla.edu/WFSRS/ASRS/asrs.html

Australasian Sleep Association (ASA):
http://bisleep.medsch.ucla.edu/WFSRS/ASA/asa.html

Austrian Sleep Research Association-ASRA
http://www.medhost.at/org/asra/

Includes a listing of Austrian sleep clinics.

Canadian Sleep Society (CSS)
http://bisleep.medsch.ucla.edu/WFSRS/CSS/css.html

"The Canadian Sleep Society / Société Canadienne du Sommeil (CSS / SCS) is a professional association of clinicians, scientists and technologists formed in June 1986 to advance education and research in sleep and its disorders in Canada."

Dutch Society for Sleep-Wake Research
http://www.socsci.kun.nl/psy/nswo/welcome.htm#NSWO

An organization for sleep research professionals in The Netherlands.

European Sleep Research Society (ESRS)
http://www.esrs.org/

"The European Sleep Research Society is an international scientific non-profit organization and promotes all aspects of sleep research. These include the publication of the Journal of Sleep Research (JSR), the organization of scientific meetings, and the promotion of training and education, the dissemination of information, and the establishment of fellowships and awards."

Finnish Sleep Research Society
http://www.utu.fi/~ollipolo/

"These pages provide information about THE FINNISH SLEEP RESEARCH ASSOCIATION and its least sleepy members. The purpose of this forum is to provide the members of the society as well as others up-to-date information about what is on for tonight in sleep research in Finland. You are likely to find out that many of us suffer from severe sleep deprivation."

German Sleep Society
http://www.uni-marburg.de/sleep/dgsm/welcome_.htm

This site includes a listing of German sleep disorder clinics.

Latin American Sleep Society
http://bisleep.medsch.ucla.edu/WFSRS/LASS/lass.html

The Sleep Research Society
http://bisleep.medsch.ucla.edu/SRS/srs_main.htm

"The Sleep Research Society exists to promote understanding of the processes of sleep and its disorders through research, the training of practitioners of research and the dissemination of the fruits of their efforts to the scientific and medical communities as well as the general public."

Society for Light Treatment and Biological Disorders
http://www.websciences.org/sltbr/

"The Society for Light Treatment and Biological Rhythms is a not-for-profit international organization founded in 1988, dedicated to fostering research, professional development and clinical applications in the fields of light therapy and biological rhythms."

Women in Sleep and Rhythm Research (WiSRR)
http://bisleep.medsch.ucla.edu/WiSRR/

"The main intention of the WiSRR group is to provide communication and mentorship between women scientists and students studying any aspects of sleep from basic science to clinical issues as they apply to both men and women."

Sleep Disorder Professionals

American Sleep Disorders Association (ASDA)
http://www.asda.org/centers.htm

Listing of accredited sleep disorder centers by state.

International Directory of Sleep Researchers and Clinicians
http://bisleep.medsch.ucla.edu/map/world.map.html

World Wide Sleep Laboratories and Clinics
http://bisleep.medsch.ucla.edu/map/world.map.html
The following is a listing of Sleep Disorder Centers or Laboratories, accredited or non-accredited reprinted from **The Sleep Medicine Home Page**, http://www.users.cloud9.net/~thorpy/.   Listing does not necessarily imply endorsement.

•AUSTRIA
•Austrian Sleep Research Association
http://www.medhost.at/org/asra/
ÖGSMSF-ASRA, PO 3, A-1145 Vienna
e-mail (asra@medhost.at)
Maintains a list of sleep disorder centers in Austria.
•Sleep Disorder Center, Pulmologic Center Vienna, Vienna, Austria •Department of Pulmonology, Elizabethinen Hospital, Linz

•AUSTRALIA
•Sleep Disorders Centre, Royal Prince Alfred Hospital, Camperdown 2050 •The Sleep Investigation Centre, North West Private Hospital Everton Park, Brisbane •The Sleep Investigation Centre, Sunnybank Private Hospital Sunnybank, Brisbane •Newcastle Sleep Disorders Centre Newcastle •Sydney Sleep Disorders Centre, Annandale, NSW •Camperdown Sleep Disorders Center, Newtown, NSW •Hornsby Sleep Disorders and Diagnostic Centre, Waitara, NSW •Satellite Sleep Laboratory, Wentworthville, NSW

•Sleep Monitoring Unit, Benowa, QLD •Central West Sleep Disorders Center, Orange, NSW •Sleep Disorders Unit, Repatriation General Hospital, Adelaide, SA •Sleep Disorders Centre, Royal Newcastle Hospital, Newcastle NSW •Sleep Disorders Centre, Austin and Repatriation Medical Centre, Heidelberg, Victoria •ACT Sleep Therapy Clinic, Deakin, Canberra •Sleep Disorders Laboratory, Malvern, Victoria •Sleep Disorders Unit, St Vincents Hospital, Darlinghurst, Sydney

•BELGIUM
•Centrum voor Stoornissen van Slapen en Waken, University Hospital, Ghent

•CANADA
•Sleep Disorders Centre, Royal Ottawa Hospital, Ottawa. •Sleep Disorders Centre of Metropolitan Toronto Toronto, Barrie, Brampton,and Richmond Hill, Canada •Sleep Insitute of Ontario, North York, Ontario •Silent Partners Sleep Clinic, Toronto •Sleep Disorders Centre, McMaster University Medical Centre, Hamilton, Ontario •The Wellesley Hospital Sleep Lab, The Wellesley Hospital, Toronto •Northern Nights Sleep Disorder Centre, Thunder Bay, Ontario •The Credit Valley Hospital Sleep Laboratory, Mississauga, Ontario

•FINLAND
Sleep Disorders Clinic and Research Center, Haaga Center for Neurological Research and Rehabilitation, Helsinki

•GERMANY
For a list of all sleep centers in Germany, contact: •German Sleep Association http://www.uni-marburg.de/sleep/ "Deutsche Gesellschaft fuer Schlafforschung und Schlafmedizin (DGSM)"

DGSM-Sekretariat, Schimmelpfengstrasse 2, 34613
Schwalmstadt-Treysa, Germany. Tel: (49)6691 2733
http://www.uni-marburg.de/sleep/•Arbeitsgemeinschaft fur ange-
wandte Schlafmedizin •Sclaflabor der Medizinschen Klinik Innen-
stadt University of munich, Munchen •Sleep Disorder Center of
Witten, Witten •Sleep Disorders Center, Regensburg •Sleep Disorders Center, Bochum

•GREAT BRITAIN
•Scottish National Sleep Center Edinburgh, Scotland. •Sleep Disorders Clinic, Leicester General Hospital, Leicester

•HONG KONG
•Sleep Assessment Unit, Department of Psychiatry, The Chinese
University of Hong Kong, Shatin NT

•IRELAND
•The Respiratory Sleep Laboratory , St. Vincent's Hospital, Elm
Park, Dublin

•ISRAEL
•The Sleep Research Unit, Sorkoa Medical Center, Beer-Seva
•Technion Sleep Laboratory, Gutwirth BLDG, Technion City,
Haifa 3200 •Sleep Disorders Unit, Lowenstein Rehabilitation Hos-
pital, Raanana •Sleep Disorders Laboratory, Tel-Aviv University,
Ramat Aviv

•ITALY
•Centre for Sleep-Related Respiratory Disorders Universita di
Roma "La Sapienza", Roma, Italy •Center for Pediatric Sleep

Disorders, Dept. Developmental Neurology and Psychiatry, University of Rome "La Sapienza", Roma

•KOREA
•Department of Neurology, Samsung Medical Center, Kangnam Ku, Seoul

•LUXEMBOURG
•Laboratoire de Sommeil , Centre Hospitalier Luxemboug

•The NETHERLANDS
•Sleep Centre Westeinde Hospital, Den Haag •Sleep Disorders Center, Hospital "de Gelderse Vallei", Ede

•NEW ZEALAND
•Southern Sleep Services, Christchurch •The Auckland Sleep Management Centre Takapuna, Auckland

•RUSSIA
•I.M.Sechenovs Institute of Evolutionary Physiology, Sankt-Petersburg

•SOUTH AFRICA
•Smith & Vermaak Sleep Laboratory, Rosepark Hospital, Bloemfontein •Division of Pulmonology, Universitas Hospital, Bloemfontein •Respiratory Clinic, Groote Schuur Hospital, Cape Town •Sleep Disorders Center, Entabeni Medical Centre North, Durban •Neurodiagnostic Laboratories, Muelmed Medical Centre, Pretoria •SleepWake Sleep Disorders Centre, Johannesburg, South Africa

•SPAIN
•Unidad del Sueno Infantil, Clinica Quiron Valencia, Valencia

•SWEDEN
•Sleep Unit, Department of Clinical Neuroscience, Sahlgren's University Hospital, Goteborg •Sleep Laboratory, Avesta Hospital, Avesta

•SWITZERLAND
•Sleep Disorders Center, HUG-Neuropsychiatry Division, 1225 Chene-Bourg

•THAILAND
•Sleep Disorders Service and Research Unit, Songkhla

•UNITED ARAB EMIRATES
•Neurology Clinic, Al Ghurair Office Tower, Dubai

•URUGUAY
•Unidad de Estudio de Trastornornos del Sueno y la Vigilia, Hospital Britanico, Montevideo

INDEX

ORDER FORM

To Order Additional Copies of
Desperately Seeking Snoozin', The Insomnia Cure from Awake to Zzzzz

Simply choose one of the following convenient ways to order:

Call Toll Free: 877-SLEEP2NITE
877-753-3726
E-Mail: order@insomniacure.com
Fax: 901-681-9269

Postal Service: Towering Pines Press, Inc.
PO Box 17923
Memphis, TN 38187
901-763-1425

Name _____

Address _____

City _____ State_____Zip_____

Telephone _____

Quantity _____

Sales Tax _____

Shipping _____

Total _____

Sales Tax:
Please add 8.25% for books shipped to Tennessee.
Shipping:
$4.00 for the first book and $2.00 for each additional book.
Payment:
_____ Check
_____ Credit Card ☐ Visa ☐ MasterCard ☐ AMEX ☐ Discover

Card Number: _____

Name on Card: _____

I understand that I may return the book(s) that I have ordered from
Towering Pines Press, Inc. for a full refund at any time-for any reason.

ORDER TODAY-TOLL FREE

ORDER FORM

To Order Additional Copies of

Desperately Seeking Snoozin', The Insomnia Cure from Awake to Zzzzz

Simply choose one of the following convenient ways to order:

Call Toll Free: 877-SLEEP2NITE
877-753-3726
E-Mail: order@insomniacure.com
Fax: 901-681-9269
Postal Service: Towering Pines Press, Inc.
PO Box 17923
Memphis, TN 38187
901-763-1425

Name _____

Address _____

City _____ State_____Zip_____

Telephone _____

Quantity _____

Sales Tax _____

Shipping _____

Total _____

Sales Tax:
Please add 8.25% for books shipped to Tennessee.
Shipping:
$4.00 for the first book and $2.00 for each additional book.
Payment:
_____ Check
_____ Credit Card ☐ Visa ☐ MasterCard ☐ AMEX ☐ Discover

Card Number: _____

Name on Card: _____

I understand that I may return the book(s) that I have ordered from
Towering Pines Press, Inc. for a full refund at any time-for any reason.

ORDER TODAY-TOLL FREE